PENGUIN BOOKS

detox

PENELOPE SACH is a practitioner of naturopathic, homeopathic and herbal medicine. She has studied in China and France, and now runs a highly successful clinic in Sydney, where she specialises in treating career professionals, sportspeople and busy homemakers whose lifestyles lead to stress and fatigue.

Penelope has developed a range of organically grown herbal tea that sells widely across Australia and Asia, and her most recent book was *The Healing Effects of Herbal Tea*.

For more about Penelope Sach, visit www.penelopesach.com.au

I DEDICATE THIS book to my loving parents,
Paula Bobbie Katherine Sach and Alan Ivens Sach,
who passed away peacefully on 16 July 2001 and
21 September 2001, respectively, while I was finishing
this book. They taught me many sound principles –
but above all they taught me to follow my dreams
and do my very best in life. I thank them for this.
May they rest in peace, joy and love.

Other titles by Penelope Sach

Natural Men's Health
The Healing Effects of Herbal Tea
Take Care of Yourself
The Little Book of Wellbeing

detox

Regaining your health and vitality

PENELOPE SACH

PENGUIN BOOKS

PENGUIN BOOKS

Published by the Penguin Group
Penguin Group (Australia)
250 Camberwell Road, Camberwell, Victoria 3124, Australia
(a division of Pearson Australia Group Pty Ltd)
Penguin Group (USA)
375 Hudson Street, New York, New York 10014, USA
Penguin Group (Canada)
10 Alcorn Avenue, Toronto, Ontario, Canada M4V 3B2
(a division of Pearson Canada Inc.)
Penguin Books Ltd
80 Strand, London WC2R 0RL, England
Penguin Ireland
25 St Stephen's Green, Dublin 2, Ireland
(a division of Penguin Books Ltd)
Penguin Group (India)
11, Community Centre, Panchsheel Park, New Delhi – 110 017, India
Penguin Group (NZ)
Cnr Airborne and Rosedale Roads, Albany, Auckland, New Zealand
(a division of Pearson New Zealand Ltd)
Penguin Group (South Africa) (Pty) Ltd
24 Sturdee Avenue, Rosebank, Johannesburg 2196, South Africa

Penguin Books Ltd, Registered Offices: 80 Strand, London, WC2R 0RL, England

First published by Penguin Books Australia Ltd 2002

9 11 13 15 16 14 12 10

Design by Susannah Low © Penguin Group (Australia)
Cover photograph by Julie Anne Renouf
Author photograph by Louise Lister
Typeset in ITC Legacy Serif by Post Pre-press Group, Brisbane, Queensland
Printed and bound in Australia by McPherson's Printing Group, Maryborough, Victoria

National Library of Australia
Cataloguing-in-Publication data:

Sach, Penelope.
Detox : regaining your health and vitality.

Bibliography.
Includes index.
ISBN 0 14 100383 9.

1. Detoxification (Health). 2. Toxins. I. Title.

615.9

www.penguin.com.au

Contents

Introduction

A DETOX PROGRAM can literally be the start of a new life. Detoxing is the essential first step in establishing a pattern of wellbeing and vitality, a pattern that should become a way of life.

The most common complaint that clients bring to me is overwhelming tiredness, chronic fatigue or a feeling of being generally 'run-down'. I hear this complaint from across the spectrum of my patients, young and old, male and female. In all cases, after taking an extensive case history and examining each particular complex of symptoms, I propose some form of simple detox program. This program may be only one or two days, or it may be three or even six weeks.

After this physical 'clean up', all of these patients report a remarkable resurgence of energy. With such a positive response to the initial detox, most of them are then physically and mentally ready to embrace an ongoing program to maintain this vitality.

Detoxification means different things to different people. Generally, we understand the word to indicate that there are toxins or poisonous substances in our systems that need to be got rid of. My role is to explain the nature of these toxins that are causing physical, and often psychological, distress; how they have developed in each patient; and how they can be eliminated. Then, we need to look at adjustments to diet and lifestyle to keep the nasties at bay.

The process of detoxification is often referred to as cleansing the body or purifying the bloodstream. Mostly my patients are aware of the presence of toxins, and will tell me: 'I just want a clean up of my body, so I can feel my old energy back and have the vitality that I felt when I was younger.' There is a wide perception that the body accumulates poisons simply from the rigours of everyday living and that we need to cleanse these toxins from the body regularly to maintain optimum wellbeing.

For centuries detoxification has been practised in varying forms. For example, Cleopatra used to bathe herself in goats' milk to maintain soft skin because women of the time realised that milk stimulates the sloughing of old skin cells to reveal a fresher complexion. The Greeks and Romans ate copious amounts of garlic, believing that it would kill all poisonous substances in the blood. Naturopaths continue to use garlic today for its powerful antiseptic properties.

From the Middle Ages, blood-letting was believed to purify the body by releasing poisons. And during the wars of the eighteenth century in England, nettles growing through the English countryside were used as a tea and rubbed on the joints externally to purify and release poisons and improve joint mobility in battle.

Now in the twenty-first century, we are still searching for new ways to purify our bodies. We are still attracted to the idea of cleansing our systems, and various fashionable methods engender countless books and articles. But one of the problems of this phase in history is that our lifestyles are so hectic. There is barely enough time to think about detoxing, let alone clearing the time to put a detox program into action. Many of us imagine wistfully that we could do some form of purification in the holiday period; but this is also a time in which we like to rest and indulge a little in the foods that we so enjoy.

After hearing about a variety of health problems from my clients, I have been able to develop ways of detoxing that can fit with relative ease into a busy lifestyle.

It's important to remember that each person has their own particular area or areas of concern. In this book, I have addressed the main problems as I have seen them in my clinical experience. You can refer to one or several areas that pertain to you, and follow the relevant detox recommendations.

If you are on any medical prescriptions, please do not undertake any detox program without first consulting your doctor or specialist.

1
Detox myths

DETOXING HAS SPAWNED a large industry. Since the '50s there have been books written on the best methods of cleansing, ranging from water fasts to juice fasts, liver cleansing diets and colonic irrigation. Forms of spiritual fasting or refraining from certain foods have been promoted to enhance body, mind and soul.

I believe that any harsh conditions imposed on the body are dangerous to your health, and unless you are under strict medical care, extreme forms of detox are unwarranted and inadvisable. In fact, my experience with detoxing has shown me that a gentle but persistent approach will yield appreciable results.

Let's look at the example of colonic irrigation, a severe detoxification method that was very much a craze in the '70s and '80s.

Under the right circumstances and control, irrigation can be useful. However, I know of several cases where this method has been completely overdone, resulting in the bowel wall losing its natural and protective flora. In this scenario, the irrigation causes painful cramps, and works against the body renewing its own superbly honed toxin defence mechanisms.

Similarly, juice fasting can generate copious amounts of sugar in the system, which can cause further problems of toxicity.

The famous Pritikin diet of the '80s eliminated all fats from the diet to avoid cardiovascular disease. History showed us that those who followed the diet felt well initially but found that their skin and hair became dry and lifeless when they followed the diet over a long period of time. Dr Pritikin later realised that natural fats in certain foods are absolutely essential for our health and wellbeing. When they were removed entirely and for the long term, skin problems escalated and heart-disease factors actually increased, because these essential fatty acids regulate the balance between 'good' and 'bad' cholesterol.

Cholesterol

Cholesterol is primarily made in the liver to carry fats around the body. High-density lipoprotein (HDL) is the 'good' cholesterol and we need to have higher amounts of this than of low-density lipoprotein (LDL), the 'bad' cholesterol, for a good medical reading. Fish oil, vegetable oils and exercise keep HDL up. LDL is increased by fried foods, a high-fat diet and diabetes and can be determined by genetics. When it is oxidised in the body, LDL becomes toxic and, further, if we do not have enough anti-oxidants in our systems, LDL becomes even more dangerous, causing a build-up of cholesterol and increasing the risk of heart disease.

Triglycerides also carry fats around the body, but they are only toxic in high doses. A diet high in refined carbohydrates such as refined sugar, lollies, fizzy drinks, white bread, pasta and alcohol will increase triglycerides. Take fish oil supplements, follow a low-fat diet and exercise regularly to keep triglycerides at an acceptable level.

case history

A forty-year-old male patient came to see me with high cholesterol, which runs in his family. Michael (I have changed his name for privacy) asked me to give him a special diet as he was determined to lower his cholesterol by natural means and exercise.

After three months he returned. He was very happy as his cholesterol levels had declined and he wanted a preventative diet to maintain this. I didn't see him then for nearly twelve months.

When he returned, he brought with him his three children for a check up. He explained that they had all suffered a lot of flus and colds during the previous winter. He also mentioned that his middle child, a girl of ten, was having learning difficulties at school and suffered from dermatitis.

After questioning, I discovered that the entire family was on a strict, no-fat regime. They were all following their father's cholesterol-lowering diet. Consequently, they had stopped eating eggs, avocados, olive oil and dairy products. This was because Michael's wife, not knowing the consequences, found it easier to cook one meal for them all, rather than one for her husband and one for the rest of the family. Neither she, nor her husband, realised that the children's diet needed to be different.

I explained the role of fatty acids in the diet, and how essential they were for growing children. Even though Michael was consuming four to six fish oil capsules a day, I cautioned him about being extreme in his diet too.

Six months later the family's diet was much more balanced. Their run of flus and colds stopped, and the dry skin of the ten-year-old improved dramatically. Also, her teachers reported a significant improvement in her reading ability and concentration.

low-fat families

It is important not to constrain children to a low-fat diet (unless they are obese and under medical supervision), as they need a varied diet of fat, carbohydrate and protein. I have often seen children suffer with dry skin, dull hair and brittle nails when they are subjected to the low-cholesterol and low-fat diets of an adult. Unsaturated fats, found in avocados, olive and canola oils and some butter, milk and cheese, are essential for growing children.

The candida (yeast-free) diet of the late '80s seemed to work for some people. However, this so-called cleansing diet was so strict and severe that many people didn't eat well or nutritionally for fear of eating the wrong thing. I remember a client on this diet coming to me. She told me that she was living on potatoes, as she was scared to eat anything else!

And then there was the raw food diet or cleanse that became popular for those who wanted to lose weight. The problem here was that many of the people who put themselves on this diet were overweight or elderly, and their digestive systems found it extremely difficult to break down and digest raw food. In fact, very young and elderly constitutions need gentle, cooked food because their digestive systems are undeveloped in the former case, and over-used and delicate in the latter.

Presently, the new-fad cleansing regime focuses on a diet high in protein and low in carbohydrate. Many people (particularly certain movie stars in the US) are calling this the wonder regime for losing weight and cleansing the system of unwanted sugars caused by excessive refined carbohydrates. Again, the individual feels better initially and can achieve quite radical weight-loss results, but staying on this regime as a maintenance program can cause and perpetuate a profound imbalance in the body.

the elderly

I do not recommend the elderly or those who are sick follow a detox program. It is too extreme for those over the age of seventy and/or those who are hospitalised. The maintenance diet can be utilised by this group and an anti-oxidant supplement is worthwhile. If you would like to modify your diet and make it healthier and anti-ageing, then it is advisable to see a naturopath to guide and assist you with any of your medication.

Doctors have always told us that a well-balanced diet is what we should aim for, but unfortunately in my experiences of consulting, many people do not really know what a well-balanced diet is. People have all sorts of ideas about what they need for optimum energy levels.

Fortunately, we now have an incredible amount of information on food. We know a lot about nutrients in foods; active elements such as anti-oxidants; enzyme-enriched foods; the basic vitamins and minerals necessary for the optimum functioning of the body: vitamins A, C and E, zinc, magnesium; and substances with names so complicated that even the scientists are flat out remembering them, let alone their chemical construction.

what is a protein?

Proteins are essential for the functioning of every organ in the body. They contain essential amino acids for building and repairing cells.

A mixture of proteins in our diet is essential and, in the past, meat protein was preferred. However, we can now choose from meat or vegetable protein. Recent research shows that vegetable protein contains isoflavones which assist in the prevention of certain forms of cancer and possibly other forms of chronic illnesses.

Animal proteins: red meat, chicken, veal, pork, eggs

Dairy proteins: milk, cheese, yoghurt

Vegetable proteins: dried pulses and legumes such as soya beans, chickpeas, lentils, broad beans, kidney beans, lima beans, split peas.

I do believe that we are in danger of being overloaded with technical information, especially through the media and the

Internet. The difficulty is that we have to understand, digest and apply the welter of data, research and statistics that changes rapidly. We have to do all this to be able to practise the principles of healthy living every day. Even as a naturopath and a medical herbalist I find the amount of professional material that appears about foods and herbs to be almost overwhelming, but it is my responsibility to translate it into practical and inspiring information for my clients.

2

What is a toxin?

A TOXIN IS a substance that is poisonous to the body. Toxins can cause minor problems such as a simple skin rash, or major ones such as cancer. In any event, toxins are harmful.

Toxins are everywhere in our daily living, from the pollution in the air we breathe to the chemicals that are formed in our bodies from the breakdown of food.

Then there are toxins from the substances that we purposely put in our bodies such as cigarette smoke, drugs – ecstasy, cocaine and heroin – and excessive alcohol, sugar, animal fats and highly processed food. Thousands of toxins are formed in the bacterial breeding ground of our large intestine, where they multiply at a rapid rate if fed a poor diet.

Toxins can breed on our food before we even consume it;

bacteria will breed on food that has been kept too long in the refrigerator; and food can ferment in heat and incorrect packaging. On the other hand, preservatives used to prevent food deteriorating can also be harmful to us when present in large doses.

Toxins are sprayed on our food in the fields to keep the bugs away. These toxins are absorbed to a greater or lesser extent into our vegetables and fruits. Toxins are formed through stress, both emotional and physical. Toxins are formed simply through being human and having a system that ages from birth to death. In fact, toxins are part of being alive. We can avoid them, remove them, minimise or neutralise them – but we need to be aware of their presence at all times. This book is about how we can adapt to toxins and survive their worst effects in the twenty-first century.

Some people believe that they can eat whatever they want, including lots of junk food, and offset the damage by taking lots of vitamins. Unfortunately, this kind of thinking is wrong, as the digestive system always prefers good nutrition. It does not wish to overload the liver with fats and sugars, and then work even harder to break down complex vitamins. The foundation of health is diet, not pills.

Others think optimum health comes from eating whatever

they like, then counteracting poisons by meditating for long hours, but the Tibetan monk who is extremely disciplined with his mind may also suffer from high blood pressure, cholesterol and major digestive disorders.

Then there are the sports-minded, who happily eat a lot of junk food and burn it up readily; but when they change their diet to take the overload off their livers and pancreases, their optimum health comes to the fore. It is interesting to note that Olympic athletes take diet very seriously to obtain that extra second or extra centimetre. Look at the way trainers feed racehorses. Only the best diet and supplements are given.

'Toxicity syndromes' are often described as a response to an overload of toxic reactions to substances that can be created internally or that enter from the external world.

Some of the familiar external toxins that we are exposed to on a daily basis are: lead from car fumes, mercury from dental amalgams, toxins from medications, pesticides from our food, preservatives and additives, detergents, household sprays, insect repellents, nail polish removers, paint thinners, industrial fumes and radiation from mobile phones.

Internal toxins are formed inside the body when it cannot process the overload. These substances are often called free radicals. Free radicals are formed naturally as part of the process of the cell using oxygen and nutrients. In a healthy individual, these are removed readily on a daily basis. But when the system is overloaded with a multiplicity of toxins, these free radicals can clump together and cause oxidative damage to the tissue. Hence we often suggest anti-oxidant supplements to assist in the removal of these free radicals and slow down the ageing process (see chapter 8).

Excessive use of refined sugar and saturated fats causes a build-up of free radicals and oxidative damage through clogging of the detox pathways of the liver (see chapter 4) and the pancreas, which is the organ metabolising the sugars in our body. Hypoglycaemia and diabetes are on the rise in our society because of the overload of junk foods we ingest regularly.

Internal toxins are formed from constipation, cigarette smoking, poor digestion and lack of oxygen. Toxins working internally can all cause major fatigue and illness and lead to cancer and heart disease.

constipation

The most common gastrointestinal complaint in the USA is constipation, and it is indicative of a diet that is too low in fibre. Unprocessed grains and legumes are the best source of fibre to assist the cleansing and detoxification of the bowel.

I have mentioned before that the body is a remarkable piece of machinery and can handle very well a certain amount of toxicity. It is when we find a conglomeration of many toxins at the same time that the body goes into serious overload. If we are exposed to toxins continuously over a period of time, then symptoms arise that reduce our quality of life.

We saw an example of this in the Gulf War. Soldiers were exposed to the anti-nerve gas agent pyristigmine bromide, the insect repellent DEET, and the insecticide permethrin. Thirteen per cent of the people involved in the war have developed neurological complaints. In a study done with hens, the individual toxins did not cause these symptoms; yet when the hens were exposed to all three toxins at the same time, neurological damage was observed.

There is still so much we do not understand about the

combined effect of toxins or what is known as 'toxic synergy'. But we do know that it is sensible to try to remove them from your environment. However, we simply have to live with some toxins. This is another reason why detoxing regularly and following the maintenance diet is useful – it helps your body to minimise the effect of the myriad toxins in our everyday lives.

3

Are you toxic?

MANY CLIENTS COME to my clinic complaining of a variation of the same problem. The words they use can be any or all of the following: 'I feel:

- tired
- fatigued
- run-down
- exhausted
- flat
- that I'm not coping well.

I feel like this a lot of the time.'

Some put their problems down to total overload in the work environment. Some blame their home atmosphere. Some feel that they are simply exhausted from the pace of the twenty-first century lifestyle. Stay-at-home parents are often suffering forms of chronic fatigue, not from a virus, but from sleep deprivation caused by the constant demand of attending to their children's needs throughout a twenty-four hour cycle, day in and day out.

Are they toxic? Maybe no, but then, maybe yes, if I delve deeper into their problems of low vitality.

sleep

Melatonin is a substance produced by the pineal gland when we go into deep sleep. It has been found that melatonin also assists in neutralising free radicals (toxins); therefore it is essential that we are not sleep-deprived. Mothers, those who travel and who suffer jet lag, and the elderly can be very run-down due to sleep disturbances. Homeopathic forms of melatonin can be obtained in Australia; in other parts of the world they are available in pharmacies.

Using an iridology torch to look into the iris of a client's eye, I find that it reveals to me several clues as to the real state of the body. The iris is like a road map, with each organ related to the iridology dial. Here, I can discern an indication of the general constitution of their body: whether their bowel is sluggish and causing excess fatigue; or whether mucus in their system is blocking lungs or breathing passageways, causing fatigue through constricted oxygen access; or whether their digestion, stomach, and/or liver is sluggish from an unhealthy diet and foods that are not breaking down efficiently to give the body the proper fuel.

Often I question patients about their stress levels. Stress puts overwhelming burdens on the adrenal glands. If these glands are overloaded, this can cause a huge upsurge in the level of exhaustion a patient experiences.

Adrenals and exhaustion

Adrenaline is a hormone sent into the blood stream from the adrenal glands when the body is under stress emotionally or physically. This hormone raises blood pressure, heart rate and sugar levels (for a quick burst of energy) and is often referred to as the 'flight and fight' hormone. Adrenaline is especially useful in times of stress, when we need to act quickly and to call on reserves of strength and endurance. These stresses can be physiological, psychological or environmental, such as sudden trauma or emergencies at work or home or even deadlines at work.

In a modern lifestyle involving a high amount of anxiety and/or stress, our adrenal glands are sending out adrenaline at too great a rate. Anecdotal evidence suggests strongly that, today, the average person is receiving around 100 stressors a day, instead of around twenty, which was average in the past. The production of this hormone is overtaxed and the glands become exhausted. This means they are unable to secrete any adrenaline at all.

This is what we refer to as 'adrenal exhaustion'. There are no reserves of adrenaline left to cope with even simple stressors such as driving a car or coping with everyday living.

Our bodies give us warning signs long before we reach adrenal overload; signs such as constant fatigue and nagging aches and pains. Ignoring these signs can lead not only to adrenal exhaustion, but to further complications such as chronic fatigue syndrome.

As a balance to stress (physical, psychological or environmental), we need to fortify the body and mind. Correct diet, supplements and exercises (such as meditation or yoga) can go far in preventing the crippling effects of adrenal overload.

Ginseng is a wonderful herb to assist adrenals under pressure.

This herb allows the glands to let out adrenaline at a more consistent rate. The glands are able to adapt more readily in times of high stress. Siberian ginseng should be taken if commencing a huge workload or gruelling sport. It is especially good for men, while women will benefit from an Indian ginseng called 'Withania'.

Liquorice root also assists the recovery of exhausted adrenals and you will find it used often in tonics to assist in rehabilitation from long-term illness.

In most cases these patients, no matter what their circumstances, improve spectacularly after a detox program. Furthermore, if they are willing to take the extra step and use the maintenance program (see chapter 6), even for 70 or 80 per cent of the time, these patients thrive. In the long run, their energy and health are maintained at much higher levels. They are happier, and feel a greater sense of wellbeing in their daily lives.

Whether you're toxic or not, detox works.

Acid and alkaline foods

Throughout history, doctors and herbalists have known the importance of keeping the blood 'balanced' for good health. We need to keep our body more alkaline than acid. Nowadays, we can read our pH levels, which should be between 7.35 and 7.45. Deviation from this can lead to illness. A great pioneer herbalist, Paavo Airola, believed that when there exists an excess of acid in the body, the acid will be deposited in joints and tissues, leading to pain in these areas. Another medical philosopher, Dr Paul Bragg, identified many symptoms associated with too much acid in the system. These include headaches, poor skin, irritability and nervous exhaustion.

The only exception to the rule of a predominance of alkalinity in a healthy system is the stomach, where acid should predominate to break down proteins. Also, our urine can be acid or alkaline depending on what is happening in the body. If our body is not eliminating waste through the bowels or kidneys efficiently, then nutritionists believe that a type of self-poisoning occurs.

The main causes of acid build-up in the digestive system are:

- poor digestion
- eating proteins and starches together frequently
- overeating meat
- excess of refined carbohydrates, including white flour and refined sugar products
- lack of fresh fruit and vegetables daily.

In today's fast-paced world of eating on the run and quick and easy meals, our diets tend to be more acidic than alkaline. When our bodies become too acidic, our system tends to use up all the reserves of minerals such as calcium, magnesium, potassium, sodium and iron. These minerals occur in high quantities in fruit and vegetables so it is critical that they are included in the diet. These minerals are essential for a healthy nervous system and for strong bones, joints and muscles. In other words, they are vital for the maintenance of a balanced temperament and for mobility.

Consult the following list to avoid too much acid, and emphasise the alkaline elements in your diet.

Acid creators
- Refined sugar and white flour products
- Meat
- Alcohol
- Stress

Alkaline creators
- Fresh fruit and vegetables
- All raw juices, especially carrot, watermelon and green vegetable juices (spinach, the top of beetroot greens and wheat grass)
- Herbal teas
- Unpasteurised honey
- Raw almonds
- Miso soup
- Tofu
- Sea vegetables
- Lima and adzuki beans (other beans, except for those which are soaked and have sprouted, are acidic)

In my detox programs, I have emphasised alkaline foods and anti-oxidants, along with some forms of protein. The overall aim is to create a well-balanced diet to enhance vitality and wellbeing.

case history

A sixty-year-old man came to me complaining of heartburn, a 'pot' stomach and sports injuries from the past in his knees and elbows.

After examining his iris, I could see that his diet was very acidic. He confirmed this by telling me that he had no breakfast except a coffee on the way to work, a business lunch generally (some form of steak or chicken with wine), followed by a takeaway dinner.

I began his treatment by asking him to drink eight glasses of water or herbal tea a day. I managed to get him to make a milkshake for breakfast, with low-fat milk, a fruit of his choice and a teaspoon of ground almonds. For his business lunches, I asked him to choose fish and two or three vegetables, three times a week; for the other two days of the working week, I allowed him to have meat (with vegetables), but required him to have a minestrone soup as entrée to 'alkalise' his system.

I supplemented his diet with a teaspoon of barley powder drink, morning and night (he wasn't fond of the taste!), and two anti-oxidant vitamins plus a vitamin B each morning after his milkshake.

Having followed this regime, he reported feeling better on his return. A lot of his aches and pains had gone (apart from his knees, which continued to trouble him) and his pot belly was not as evident.

At this stage, I prescribed two magnesium tablets in the morning to help his sugar balance and high acid levels and asked him to drink a large carrot and celery juice every day at afternoon tea. This was easy for him, as his secretary bought one daily, close by.

By the time of his second visit, he reported a great upsurge in his health and vitality. He was back playing eighteen holes of golf, and his joints and knees seemed to be holding up very well.

Do you need to detox?

Read the following list.

If you have three or more of the following symptoms then a three-day detox will improve your health and wellbeing, especially if you follow the detox with the maintenance diet (see chapter 6).

- Fatigue
- Lethargy
- Moodiness
- Irritability
- Sleeplessness
- Anxiety
- Vagueness
- Poor memory
- Poor concentration
- Stomach aches
- Bloated stomach
- Indigestion
- Sluggish bowel
- Blocked nose
- Excessive mucus
- Sore muscles

- Aching joints
- Blotchy skin
- Itchy skin
- Persistent skin problems
- Pimples
- Bad breath
- Furry tongue

Now consider this next list. Are any of the following featuring prominently in your lifestyle?

- Pollutants from cars, factories and city living
- Radiation from mobile phones
- Pollens and grasses
- Cleaning agents and washing detergents
- Dust mites
- Poisonous baits
- Preservatives and additives in your diet
- Colourings in your food
- Refined sugar in your diet: fizzy drinks,
  lollies and sweets
- High coffee intake
- Restaurants

- High-fat diet
- Alcohol
- Cigarettes
- Recreational drugs: marijuana, ecstasy, cocaine, heroin
- Prescription drugs: codeine, anti-inflammatories, antibiotics, sleeping pills, laxatives, anti-depressants
- Surgery or hospitalisation
- Stress
- Depression
- Insomnia
- A sedentary job
- Shift work
- Late nights
- Global travel
- Illness related to age
- Cholesterol
- Excess weight
- Yeast infections
- Smelly teeth, hands, feet
- Sexual problems
- Headaches

- Repeated viruses: glandular fever, herpes, shingles, influenza
- Red, sore and swollen eyes

If the answer is yes, you should look at detoxing and following a maintenance program.

When NOT to Detox

- During pregnancy
- If you suffer from major heart disease
- If you are over seventy-five or under twelve
- When you are on prescribed medication (check with your doctor)
- If you are under extreme pressure emotionally or physically (training for a sports competition, for example; or if you are recovering from the loss of a loved one)
- If you are significantly underweight

While the factors listed mean that you should not detox, you will be able to follow the maintenance diet with enthusiasm. This diet will work over a period of time, providing you persist, and give you more vitality and a heightened sense of wellbeing.

Consult your naturopath for suitable supplements for individual conditions or factors.

Which detox do I start with?

If you're feeling a bit run down and needing just a bit more vim and vigour in your life, you probably need a general detox. The detox for food substances is the most general detox, especially if followed by the maintenance diet (see chapter 6).

Otherwise choose the detox that's related to your individual health requirements. For instance, just before winter, try the detox for lungs and respiratory tract.

How often should I detox?

Do a three-day detox three times a year, particularly as a springboard into a healthier lifestyle e.g. after Christmas, before winter and in spring.

Note: You should not detox when you are sick, because it lowers your immune system too much.

4

Natural detox systems

THE BODY HAS its own ways of detoxing naturally. Let's put this simply. The liver acts as a purifying filter for the blood. The gall bladder assists the liver and also breaks down fats. The kidneys eliminate unwanted elements (such as excessive uric acid, proteins and bacteria) in our body. The bowel eliminates unwanted waste, bacteria and toxins from the breakdown of our foods. Without these systems working properly together, we would be walking toxic bombs. We would suffer toxaemia (blood poisoning) very quickly and become prey to other life-threatening diseases.

Normally, we take these bodily functions for granted. We

don't have to think about them much. However, when we undertake a detox program we tend to become more aware of how our body is operating. As we start to feel better, we become tuned into the vital role these organs play in health and wellbeing.

Let's look at the liver first, as it plays a critical role in keeping our bodies toxin-free.

The liver

For centuries, various cultures have referred to the liver as the 'cleansing' organ of the body. It is also the largest organ. These two facts combined mean that we must treat the liver with some respect. Taken to the extreme, the human body cannot survive for more than twenty-four hours without an adequately functioning liver.

One of the basic rules in naturopathic and herbal medicine (a rule that has been passed on for centuries and is now proven with modern methods) is that many illnesses can be treated by enhancing and assisting liver function.

Various physical signals will alert us to toxin overload in the liver. Problems with the liver may cause bad temper. The whites of the eyes may turn yellowish. After even one heavy night out with alcohol, our eyes will look 'boiled', and we will experience that seedy feeling of 'toxicity'.

Other signs of toxic overload on the liver are: dark circles under the eyes; a sallow skin colour; headaches; a yellow-coated tongue; irritability; PMS; joint problems; skin rashes; inability to digest fats; indigestion; nausea; and often a general feeling of malaise combined with sluggishness.

The primary function of the liver is to filter and detoxify our blood. This process removes harmful toxins such as bacteria, viruses, yeasts, toxic poisons and any other foreign substances, such as pharmaceuticals; contaminated food; pesticides; heavy metals; and pollution and chemicals in the home environment. A well-functioning liver will also remove substances that cause allergies.

In the process of cleansing, the liver also performs a number of other critical bodily functions:

- It helps to metabolise and regulate the levels of protein, fats and carbohydrates.
- It regulates the levels of triglycerides and cholesterol.
- It also plays an important part in the storage of vitamin A and D, B_{12} and iron.

How does the liver detoxify? Basically, it is a highly sophisticated plumbing system. When overload occurs, think of a blockage in your sink: there's a back-surge of unwanted material. Generally, however, the organ is able to take a lot of overload because there are two main detoxification systems, and they cover one another. The first system processes the blood very rapidly, leaving further breaking down to the second system. Imagining the liver as a great plumbing network is to understand and appreciate the effect of too many poisons and toxins. It just cannot filter them out as quickly as they are taken in.

The first filtering stage in the liver slows down with ageing and the use of pharmaceutical medication, including oral contraceptives. Exposure to lead, mercury and cadmium (from cigarette smoking) and the overuse of refined sugar and saturated fats can also make first-stage filtering very sluggish.

Sometimes the opposite can happen. Where the first-stage toxins are broken down too rapidly, there can be an overload on the second stage, which cannot keep up. Poisons that are not broken down completely are released into the bloodstream as free radicals, which can cause major diseases of the brain, liver and immune system. Substances that are known to cause the first stage to accelerate too rapidly are pesticides, paint fumes, cigarettes, alcohol and steroids (especially when these toxins are combined with each other or with prescription medicine, for example).

Diet is the key to maintaining a healthy liver and the benefits of wellbeing and vitality. The liver must be supported with the following foods to enhance the two main stages of detoxification:

- vegetables such as cabbage, broccoli, turnips, brussel sprouts, celery, onions, horseradish, watercress, string beans, kale and soyabeans, which contain natural sulphur
- proteins such as eggs, fish and meat, which are also excellent sources of sulphur.

Nutritionally, these foods are vital for the 'sulfation pathways' in the liver which assist in breaking down steroid hormones, prescription and recreational drugs, industrial chemicals, compounds from plastics, disinfectants and toxins from the bacteria in our intestine and the environment.

Certain fatty acids (omega 3 and 6 oils) are important in the first phase of the detox process. These are present in cold-water fish such as salmon and tuna, and flaxseed oils. Other foods that contain these substances are cold-pressed oils from sunflowers and walnuts, evening primrose oil, wheat germ oil and sesame seed oil. These oils should be used raw and not cooked.

Essential fats

Omega 3 and omega 6 essential fatty acids are pure, or unsaturated, fats. Omega 3 is found in high concentrations in oily fish such as salmon, halibut, mackerel, sardines and tuna. Omega 6 is found in high concentrations in vegetable sources such as evening primrose, canola, sunflower and safflower oils, and in lower concentrations in olive and almond oils.

Both groups are essential for brain development in children. There has been a link with deficiencies of omega 3 and omega 6 and incidences of Attention Deficit Disorder. When given supplements of these essential fatty acids, boys, in particular, had less temper tantrums, less headaches and less stomach problems. Supplements were also shown to assist children who suffered asthma, hayfever, other allergies and eczema.

The vegetable oils should always be used in first-press, cold-press form to gain maximum medicinal value. Alternatively, take capsules, particularly when prescribed by your naturopath.

These essential fatty acids are also vital for lowering 'bad' cholesterol (LDL) and assisting the function of 'good' cholesterol (HDL). They also nourish joints and assist joint problems (see chapter 11).

Certain herbs powerfully assist both stages of cleansing. They are:

- tumeric
- sage
- rosemary
- garlic
- sassafras
- caraway seeds
- dill seeds.

Nutrients that assist, especially in the first stage of the liver process, are:

- folic acid
- vitamin B_{12}
- selenium
- green tea
- schisandra
- St Mary's thistle
- glycine
- choline
- cystine
- taurine
- methionine.

Silybum marianum, or St Mary's thistle, has the
incredible effect of drawing out chemicals from
tissue, particularly liver tissue, where many poisons
accumulate. This herb can be taken as a bitter tea or
as a tablet after you have eaten an orange vegetable,
as this plant works especially well in this combination.
Fruits can be a little too acidic when combined with
the strong detoxing attributes of the herb. Try half a
tablet at first as you may feel a little nauseated on
full strength.

I often advise my patients to take this herb after
their lunch to give their liver a chance to detox after
being up and about for five to six hours.

Citrus fruits replenish glutathione, a substance vital for the
second stage of detoxification.

Nutrients that assist especially in the second phase are:

- niacin
- vitamin B_2
- vitamin C.

The gall bladder

This organ lies just beneath the liver and is like a catching system for the toxins that have somehow missed the liver-detox system, or are only partly detoxed. We can tell something is wrong here when we feel generally unwell and headachy. More serious gall bladder problems are indicated when we vomit up bile or are diagnosed with gallstones. Gallstones are created when the gall bladder fails to process efficiently.

The liver excretes its toxins in the form of a liquid called bile, which runs into the gall bladder and from there into the intestine. Bile consists of cholesterol, lecithin and a substance called bilirubin, with some toxins.

Bile is used by the intestine to continue the breaking down of fats. However, if bile is processed inefficiently by the gall bladder then stones and bile salts are formed. These stones block the further breaking down of fats, causing digestive pain, headaches, nausea and sometimes vomiting.

A diet high in vegetables and low in saturated fat and refined sugars will help to prevent these problems.

You can assist the gall bladder by:

- eating lecithin (500 gm supplements), which helps to keep the bile flowing and prevent the formation of stones
- including soluble fibre, such as the pectin in raw apples and other fruits, or oat bran in your diet
- drinking dandelion root tea daily
- eating small meals, frequently
- sipping on the juice of half a lemon in warm water daily
- increasing omega 3 and 6 oils (see page 40).

The kidneys

The kidneys are responsible for ridding the body of excess toxic substances through urination. Good hydration is critical to the healthy functioning of the kidneys. The rule for hydration under normal circumstances is drinking eight glasses of purified water on a daily basis, and up to two litres a day when on a detox program.

Clients who are dehydrated report that their urine becomes concentrated in colour and emits a pungent smell. The urine of a body that is properly hydrated will have a sweeter smell and a much lighter colour. I also observe that those patients who drink very little are particularly fatigued and often complain of kidney pain.

When kidney pain is a symptom, a doctor can test the urine for bacteria, excess protein and other toxic substances that can cause urinary tract infections and also kidney stones. It is vital that clients who have been diagnosed with kidney stones (whether of uric acid or calcium) make a concerted effort to drink water or herbal teas regularly. Good hydration will keep the concentrations of these stones to a minimum and assist in flushing them out if they are small enough in size.

cranberry juice

Cranberries contain a unique phytonutrient especially beneficial to the urinary tract. They are a natural cleanser for the kidneys, and prevent and relieve the symptoms of urinary tract infections, especially in the elderly.

The intestinal tract

Simply put, this is a long tube which runs from your mouth to the end of your large intestine. The intestine has hundreds of small inlets called 'villi' that allow the surface of the small and large intestine to be hundreds of times larger than its length to allow for total reabsorption of vital nutrients.

The intestinal tract is really a remarkable piece of machinery. To think that our food is sometimes thrown into our mouths without much thought!

The large and small intestine, often referred to as the bowel, can breed many microscopic forms of bacteria. The bowel is host to a wealth of 'good' bacteria, which help in the processing of foods. This is our natural intestinal flora. However, through poor diet and the use of drugs, particularly antibiotics, the bowel can breed thousands of 'bad' bacteria, which throw the natural balance out of sync. It is important that the natural balance of good and bad bacteria is restored in the intestine. Through the continual replacement of the good bacteria with lactobacillus and lacto bifidus, found in yoghurt (and if needed in larger therapeutic doses, through a supplement of powder or capsule), equilibrium is maintained.

The inner lining of the intestinal tract is referred to as a mucous membrane. This membrane takes all sorts of bumps and knocks as food passes down the tract and is processed by many enzymes on the way, from the salivary glands to the liver, the pancreas, and the small and large intestines. The inner lining has come under much scientific scrutiny in the last decade. Scientists have been exploring the integrity of the wall, and how toxins can be absorbed back through a breach in the wall, into the bloodstream, where they cause oxidative damage. This damage affects other organs including the kidneys, the brain and, of course, the liver. Hostile bacteria that sit in the bowel over a long period of time (nourished by poor diet and little fibre) lead to putrefaction. This creates a breeding ground for further bad bacteria to multiply, which, in turn, causes damage to the wall, and also allows the bad bacteria to be reabsorbed back through the breach.

When the lining of the intestine becomes damaged, our body begins to break down, showing symptoms of lowered immunity, bloating and gas, inconsistent stools, bleeding from the bowel or acute and chronic pain in these areas.

Scientists are now referring to this syndrome as 'a leaky gut' or 'intestinal permeability'. We see clear cases of leaky gut syndrome in Crohn's disease, food allergies, coeliac disease (intolerance to gluten from all grains except rice), rheumatoid arthritis and schizophrenia.

Intestinal permeability increases with age. So as we age, it is important to follow sensible dietary and supplementary programs to maintain the health of our intestinal tract.

gluten

Some people are gluten-intolerant, or intolerant to a protein in grains (wheat, barley, rye and oats) that causes inflammation of the wall of the intestine and acts like a severe 'toxin'. This protein is not present in rice. Check with your doctor or health consultant for symptoms and specific tests.

Inflammation of the lining is common to most bowel problems. Unfortunately, anti-inflammatory drugs can further exacerbate the irritation of the wall, so it is vital to eat gentle, reparative foods to promote healing (see chapter 11).

Naturopathic practitioners have always been aware that digestion and reabsorption of the right nutrients – and not toxic substances – are the key to ongoing vitality.

A detox program is vital to begin any repair of the mucous membrane of the intestine, and to rid the body of food intolerances that may be causing minor toxicity problems.

The repair of the intestinal walls and membranes takes time and patience. By using the detox and maintenance sections and being vigilant about diet and lifestyle, the benefit will be a great increase in your vitality and the ability of your body to heal.

5

Detox – how it works

I LOOK AT detox as a process that only starts with the initial rigorous clean out. The detox process for each particular complaint is divided into three main sections.

The first section is a description of the three-day procedure for each particular problem. When you decide to detox, try to choose three days when you are not working, or a long weekend.

There are a number of points to remember about the three-day detox:

- No alcohol, cigarettes or other pollutants should interfere with this critical stage.
- No vitamins are to be taken in the detox unless stated. If you feel constipated, then a teaspoon of vitamin C

powder can be taken in a glass of water three times a
day; or a teaspoon of pysillium husks twice a day; or a
teaspoon of vegetable oil two or three times a day.

- Remember that the worst period is usually in the first
  forty-eight hours. After this period, you can expect to
  feel a renewed vigour.
- Less frequently, muscle and joint pain can occur.
  Occasionally, my patients report skin breakouts. In a
  three-day cleanse these issues are usually minor. Know
  they will pass, and look forward to the renewed energy
  after the hard work.

Secondly, I talk about the wellbeing stage, which is roughly the
six-week phase after the three-day clean out. This is possibly the
most important part of the detox process. You have managed to
discipline yourself for the initial cleanse, and now you need to use
this achievement as a springboard to inspire and motivate you
into a continued state of good health. I call this the wellbeing
stage because you will have a feeling of greater vitality, a clearer
mind and a more evenly balanced temperament. These are the
results of a successful first-stage detox, and these results can
continue if you follow the advice in this second section.

Thirdly, I discuss supplementation for each particular problem. These are the vitamin and mineral supplements that should be taken during the wellbeing phase, and as a maintenance program afterwards to keep in top shape.

But, ultimately, the detox process is only as good as its maintenance. This means that once the detox process is through, you will need to look at maintaining a healthy approach to your diet and your environment to continue to reap the rewards. The key words here are consistency and frequency. I will help you to map a path to suit your needs so that staying healthy is effortless, even for those with the most hectic of lifestyles. (See the maintenance diet, chapter 6.)

If you are not feeling mentally ready to start immediately on a three-day detox, you may prefer to start with the more general maintenance diet. Once you have adapted this program to your everyday living, you should have much more energy. You will discover how much your health has improved by committing to a basic regular, healthy eating pattern. You may then decide to start on one of the detoxes. The main thing is to listen to your body and do what feels right for you, especially in relation to your lifestyle, work commitments and time management.

What can I eat?

The rigours of the three-day detox should not be overwhelming. I have devised several basic recipes for broths, soups and juices, which can be used for the detox programs and also during the maintenance diet. These recipes can be adjusted slightly depending on the specific detox and the time of year. Often, I recommend that you consume soup for the whole three days; however, in summer you may prefer to make a smoothie or a fresh juice, alternating occasionally with some soup. Use the recipes on pages 162–168 as a guide to how to prepare simple sustenance.

What to expect in a detox

During a detox, the liver is working at a steady speed to rid the body of toxins and often you can experience some nausea or a feeling of being 'off colour' for the first few days. Water must be a high priority. Sip on room-temperature water, approximately a glass every hour, to help the flushing out of toxins through the liver, kidneys and intestines. Ginger tea can assist when you experience nausea. Sipping on lemon juice in water is helpful to the gall bladder if there is any unusual vomiting. If vomiting persists, you should see your doctor.

If you experience any sharp pains or a continual pain that persists over several days in the lower back, drink copious amounts of water in case the kidneys have small stones which they are trying to pass. If severe pain persists, it is advisable to check with your doctor for stones that could have been lodged for a number of years and need to be passed in a hospital.

Some bloating and wind is quite common due to cleaning of the wastes and bacteria that ferment in the bowel. Capsules of acidophilus and bifidus can be taken to reduce this unpleasantness, usually one to two before each main meal. If you are not allergic to lactose, then take an acidophilus yoghurt tablet two to three times a day, half an hour before eating or an hour after eating.

Charcoal tablets can be taken if the bowel is sluggish and very 'windy'. One tablet after each main meal helps to absorb unwanted gases and toxins. A teaspoon full of psyllium husks or a teaspoon of cold-pressed vegetable oil after each meal can alleviate constipation.

Some people can experience diarrhoea and if this is the case, do not allow the body to become dehydrated. Keep up your fluid intake and eat a banana (to replace lost potassium – see below) and include some rice to 'bind' the excessive diarrhoea. If it persists for several days, it should be checked by a doctor to make sure you have not picked up a virus or some bacteria that need to be killed through the use of an antibiotic. Sometimes parasites give rise to these symptoms, and a stool check with your doctor is appropriate.

As more fluids are drunk, urination becomes more frequent. This is to be expected. More frequent urination can cause a drop in the body's potassium levels. For those on blood pressure medication, check with your doctor about potassium loss. Bananas can be eaten after the detox program to restore potassium, or a mineral tablet can be prescribed to take during the detox if necessary.

Bowel motions may be loose. For those who have suffered sluggish bowel movements, elimination is generally greatly improved.

After completing any detox program, it is important to include yoghurt with the healthy bacteria acidophilus, and/or acidophilus powder or tablets, in the diet. These foods soothe and reline the bowel wall and assist in breaking down food in this organ. Take one small pot of this yoghurt daily or a teaspoon of the powder before each meal.

Fibre is important. Fibre can be included in your diet with raw salads; or sprinkle a teaspoon of psyllium on your cereal in the morning or dissolve it in a glass of water in the evening.

Fibre

Fibre acts as a carrier to move and dispel wastes in the intestine. It does not break down in the processing of other foods and nutrients and is often referred to as an insoluble cellulose material. Without enough fibre, we suffer constipation and a build-up of bad bacteria in our faeces.

The best fibre comes from the outside of wholemeal grains, the skin on apples and pears (with the fruit also), the pith on oranges and the fibre in raw celery, carrots and psyllium husks. Importantly, adequate amounts of fibre in the diet prevent bowel cancer, as fibre keeps the bowel dispelling toxins that would otherwise build up over years and cause oxidative damage.

It is interesting to note here that tribes from areas in Africa and South America and the top of India, known as Hunzaland, who eat a high-fibre diet with fruits and vegetables and no refined products, have far less incidence of bowel cancer than those of us on the typical Western diet, filled with refined foods, preservatives and additives.

Food intolerance and the bowels

In my practice I see many children who suffer from poor bowel movements. Many of them are shy of discussing this problem with their parents or teachers. The first sign is usually persistent complaints from the child about stomach aches. These children can be subject to major food intolerances that block passageways, and they need to be monitored subtly.

I do not encourage children to go on a detox program, but monitored by a naturopath or doctor, food intolerances can be diagnosed and slowly eliminated from the diet. Healthier foods, suitable for the needs of the individual child, can be gradually incorporated, replacing foods that are intolerable to their system.

With adults, unless food intolerances are treated (I advise patients to keep a daily diary of food intake for two to three weeks to assist in the diagnosis of this condition), then irritable bowel syndrome will occur with all its attendant problems of discomfort and long-term fatigue. A detox is especially important here. Ideally, the maintenance diet must then be followed, leaving out any foods that regularly spark diarrhoea or constipation.

It has been found those children and adults with Attention Deficit Disorder or some form of hyperactivity often suffer from 'leaky gut' syndrome (see pages 47–48). This syndrome describes a dysfunctional process whereby toxins from food and those absorbed from the environment (such as fumes, pollution and even some perfumes) leak through the bowel wall into the surrounding cell membrane. This leaking causes a form of toxaemia in the surrounding healthy cells. In turn these toxic substances irritate all the other organs of the body. Symptoms such as irritability, fatigue, poor concentration, moodiness and irrational behaviour are common.

6
The
maintenance diet

THERE IS NO point in committing yourself to the discipline and the motivation of the detox program unless you continue to follow a well-balanced diet after the initial three-day detox. The maintenance diet should become a way of life that continues to build on the positives of the detox program without the extreme of eliminating toxins at such a fast rate.

Unfortunately many people feel so well during the three-day detox program that they continue on it for far too long. This can cause serious reverse effects because the body needs a balanced diet and fuel to thrive and grow.

Remember that a detox program is used to speed up the

elimination of toxins and is to be used for a short time only.

A repair state after the initial removal of toxins is vital for continued health. The maintenance program revolves around a continued state of daily elimination of toxins and the ongoing repair of tissues. This diet focuses on a balance of quality protein, quality carbohydrates and fruits and vegetables high in anti-oxidants. It is as essential to everyday life as walking and talking.

To begin the day

Drink a glass of filtered water, at least 300 ml. Warm water with the juice of half a lemon is ideal for those with liver or mucus problems.

Breakfast

Choose one of the following:

🌿 Two pieces of wholemeal toast with one to two boiled or poached eggs.

eggs

Eggs are a high-quality protein, rich in minerals, iron, B vitamins and an important nutrient called lecithin, essential for the development of brain nerve pathways. Small amounts of cholesterol are present in the egg yolk but recent research suggests that small amounts of cholesterol in food does not cause a problem if you are consuming a diet that is low in saturated fats such as butters, cheeses and fried foods.

Two eggs every second day are ideal for adults and children. Eggs give complete protein and energy for the day, and are especially good for children, contributing to growth and energy reserves.

🍀 Two slices of wholemeal toast with a protein snack such as herrings, sardines, tuna or salmon. Note: This is a good source of protein as well as omega 3 and 6 oils for those with cholesterol and any dry skin problems.

🍀 A muesli with a mixture of wholemeal grains, finely ground nuts and naturally dried fruit, with low-fat milk or soya milk. Note: this is excellent for those with sluggish digestive systems and gives sustained energy for a number of hours. Not recommended for those with allergies to dried fruit, such as asthmatics and candida sufferers.

* A light cereal such as Weet-Bix with low-fat milk or soya milk, followed by a slice of wholemeal toast with some form of protein; for example, tinned fish, baked beans, egg, tahini paste or low-fat white cheese. Note: This breakfast gives fibre and energy for the morning with protein to repair and feed cell tissue.

* A fruit salad with a high-quality yoghurt with acidophilus bacteria. To follow, a small snack of carbohydrate with protein; for example, a piece of wholemeal toast with a spread of almond butter or tahini paste or a high-quality fish paste. Vegemite can be used if you have no allergies to yeast products.

* A protein milkshake made with low-fat milk or soya milk with added protein powder and fruit of your choice. Lecithin powder, wheat germ powder and ground nuts can be added with or without the protein powder. Yoghurt is

ideal for its healthy bacteria and either dairy or soya milk yoghurt can be used (two teaspoons in the milkshake).

❀ A wholemeal porridge with a protein over the top such as ground almonds, yoghurt and/or milk. This is ideal in colder weather.

Fluids to accompany breakfast:
- A glass of freshly squeezed orange juice. Do not use bottled juice.
- A glass of freshly squeezed orange and pineapple juice. Especially useful for those wanting to continue the detox of the lungs.
- A freshly squeezed carrot and ginger juice. This is especially useful for those with sluggish livers and digestive systems. It does not mix well if it is drunk too close to other breakfast foods. Ideally, drink it 45 minutes before eating other foods. If this is difficult, take the juice to work and drink it one hour later.
- A cup of black tea or green tea for anti-oxidant levels or herbal tea for your specific problem areas (see pages 169–172).

Morning tea

Choose one of the following:

🍀 A large carrot and ginger juice, or orange and pineapple juice, or a jug of filtered water on your desk with freshly squeezed or sliced lemon in the water.

🍀 One to two pieces of fresh fruit.

🍀 Herbal tea to taste.

🍀 A light snack if you are following through the detox on sugar, smoking, or irregular eating habits that have caused anxiety and nervous symptoms. One of the following can be chosen:
- One to three wholewheat biscuits or rice crackers with a protein on top. This will help you control the cravings for sugar and junk foods without gaining weight. It also assists the body to burn excess toxins.
- A high-quality yoghurt with one fruit.
- A small handful of nuts with dried fruit. Not suitable for those with an allergy to nuts or dried fruit.

- A protein low-fat milkshake (obtainable from a quality health food store). A fruit can be added.

Lunch

Choose one of the following:

❧ A wholemeal sandwich with a protein and one of each of the coloured vegetables – orange, white and green.

vegetables by colour

You can often tell the properties of vegetables by their colour. For example, orange vegetables such as carrot, pumpkin and sweet potato are good anti-oxidants, as are the white vegetables potato, cauliflower and cucumber. Green vegetables – spinach, rocket, lettuce and parsley – are excellent sources of iron and chlorophyll.

❧ A wholemeal rice salad with a protein and three different vegetables, raw or cooked, in three different colours. Not fried rice.

🍀 A Japanese meal consisting of sushi followed by a protein of beef or chicken teppanyaki or tofu with a salad.

p r o t e i n s   a r e :
tuna, salmon and other fish, eggs, chicken, beef, legumes, tofu, white cheese (cottage, ricotta or fetta), a tahini or nut spread. (See also page 12.)

🍀 A thick vegetable soup with beef, chicken, fish or legumes. Add a slice of wholemeal bread or toast if you have no food intolerance to yeast or are not trying to lose excess kilos.

Vegetarians can use as protein legumes such as lentils, chickpeas, soya beans, lima beans, split peas or a variety of nuts with the three different vegetables – orange, white and green. They can also have tofu or white cheese.

🍀 Egg noodle soup with three coloured vegetables and a protein.

🌺 A protein, grilled or casseroled, with a selection of the three coloured vegetables. Note: this is very appropriate when dining in a restaurant at lunchtime.

🌺 You should always include vegetable juices, which are better with a vegetable and protein lunch than fruit juices. Water can dilute your digestive enzymes when eating and cause some bloating and discomfort. Ideally, use fluids moderately and drink an hour before or after eating.

🌺 You may drink wine during a meal – in moderation – as it assists digestion.

Afternoon snack

🌺 A fruit or a yoghurt or both.

🌺 A crispy biscuit with a spread of a protein (see morning tea snack). This is appropriate for those coming off sugar and cigarette smoking or for those who are moody and have irregular eating habits.

🦋 A raw vegetable juice or fruit juice

🦋 A handful of almonds or other nuts but not peanuts for those with liver troubles.

Dinner

Choose one of the following:

🦋 A protein from page 66, grilled, in a casserole or baked. Choose three coloured vegetables, preferably 50 per cent cooked and 50 per cent as a raw salad.

🦋 A rice dish with a protein and three coloured vegetables. Salad on the side.

🦋 A pasta with a protein; for example, bolognaise or seafood sauce (use cream sauces very moderately). Thai or curry spices with meat or fish could be used as a sauce with egg noodles.

🍀 A legume dish with a variety of beans – chickpeas, soya beans and kidney beans – mixed with sautéed vegetables and a spice such as ginger, chilli or garlic, or all three.

🍀 For dessert, have some fresh fruit salad or stewed fruit and yoghurt. Stewed fruit is excellent for those with bowel problems, a weak digestive system or sugar cravings.

Supper

🍀 A yoghurt or a glass of soya milk, cow's milk or rice milk. Add some honey if you are craving sweetness.

totally avoid the following:

Junk foods

Fizzy drinks

Cordials

Highly coloured sweets

Cigarettes

Recreational drugs

avoid the following (or have very occasionally):

Fried foods

Rich sauces with added creams

Highly processed tinned foods

Preservatives, additives and colourings

Processed meat products

Refined sugar – cakes and sweet biscuits

Refined white flour products including white bread
and white pasta

7

Detox for food substances

I BELIEVE THE consistent overuse of certain food substances is one of the most depleting and disturbing hazards to our health. What are these substances? How do they work in our body? And how do we assist our body to get rid of them?

Firstly, there are substances such as sugar that we ingest in very unbalanced proportions. These substances overload our systems and can cause a breakdown in our actual tissue or cell structures. This breakdown causes imbalances in our body with the long-term effect of poor health and/or disease, which, with a little education, conscious effort and daily good habits, could be avoided in many cases.

Secondly, there are substances such as colourings, preservatives and additives. Most consumers are aware of the presence of these ingredients, but it is often difficult to control our intake. They are used in many forms and are, to some extent, part and parcel of the food we eat.

Let's deal with one of the most obvious dietary overloads first: refined sugar.

Sugar

The most abused food substance in our society is refined sugar. I am not talking about a moderate use of refined sugar here. I am referring to the total sugar overload of which many of us are unaware. Refined sugar is hidden in many foods. It can cause a slow, inexorable breakdown of tissue and organs. It also plays havoc with our children's diet and their general behaviour. Sugar ferments with other food in our bowel and can cause bacteria to breed and multiply rapidly, especially in the presence of yeasty substances such as bread, cheese and alcohol.

Simple physical symptoms of sugar abuse are fatigue, irritability, mood swings, insomnia, and an inability to concentrate for long periods at a time without a sugar intake. Other symptoms include itchy skin and aching joints, and, of course, a craving for regular sugar 'hits'.

Foods to be aware of:
- lollies of all sorts
- fizzy drinks
- chocolate
- ice-cream
- alcohol
- fruit in large amounts
- cakes
- sweet biscuits
- cordials
- tinned sugary foods
- white bread, white pasta and white rice.

These foods will often also carry large amounts of colourings and preservatives.

It is not a good idea to go cold turkey and stop all sugars in your diet at the same time. This can be dangerous and counter-productive. Your body can go into a type of shock, and you can be overwhelmed with worse fatigue than you have ever felt in your life.

If you suspect you are overloaded with sugar, keep a diary for two weeks, meticulously recording your food intake. (Remember, you are only cheating yourself if you leave something out.) If you are showing sugar overload symptoms, and you find that you are ingesting sugar several times through the day, then you are ready for a sugar detox.

Sugar detox procedure

To clean out sugar from your system, it would be incorrect to overload the body with concentrated, naturally occurring sugars, such as those in fruit and raw vegetables. The ideal basis for your sugar detox is an alkaline cleanse made from cooked vegetables in the form of soup. It is gentle and bland: it will absorb excess sugar build-up in the blood stream, and it will heal nerves frayed by stress.

The reason these soup broths work so well in sugar detox, as well as other forms of detox related to the nervous system and joints, is that they are naturally high in minerals such as magnesium, potassium and other trace elements. These alkaline minerals soothe, protect and feed the system without the acidic effects of the refined sugar and the concentrated sugars in fruit (see acid and alkaline foods, pages 25–29).

Stage one: 3 day detox

🍀 Make a soup broth of parsley, onions, carrots, turnips, zucchini, broccoli and cauliflower (see pages 162–163). The vegetables can be eaten (immediately, or mashed up in soup) or simply sieve the fluid off and drink it.

🍀 Drink only two glasses of raw carrot juice during the day (carrots can be quite high in sugar), mixed with beetroot or a green vegetable such as spinach or lettuce.

🍀 If you crave fruit, then eat a whole piece every alternate hour from the soup. The only fruits allowed are an orange, apple or pear.

🍀 Drink a large bowl or cup (at least 300 ml) of soup every two hours of your waking day. Follow this procedure for three days.

🍀 Drink pure spring or filtered water in between the soup so that two litres of water are consumed per day (on top of the consumption of the soup).

🍀 Drink a glass of water every hour to keep the body cleansed from the overload of sugar in your system.

🍀 Rest for at least two hours a day. Only light walking is recommended during the detox.

🍀 During this detox stage you may feel some form of headache, fatigue, weakness in the limbs, or mental vagueness.

🍀 If you feel too headachy, eat steamed vegetables every three hours to give you a more alkaline effect from the detox.

You may wish to take some minor supplements if you are struggling (see stage three).

Stage two: wellbeing

Now that you have cleaned out some of the overload of the sugar in your body it is critical that you develop a regime that eliminates most refined sugars and other sugars from your diet. Maintain this program for about six weeks and be sure to include supplementation as necessary (see stage three).

- Do not buy or eat any food that is refined or processed, such as white sugar, fizzy drinks, cordials, chocolates, sweets, puddings or desserts.

- Avoid hidden sugars found in tinned food, sweet milks, processed yoghurt, sweetened tea and coffee, jams and preserves.

- Food and snacks need to be taken regularly in short and small bursts for at least six weeks until the body becomes used to metabolising more efficiently.

Here is an easy guide:
- Eat a piece of fresh fruit every time you would like to eat refined sugar.

- Eat fruit in between meals, especially stoned fruit, to stop the habit of reaching for sweets and chocolates in the afternoon.
- Replace white bread and white rice with wholemeal bread and, where possible, wholemeal rice. You could be adventurous and try other grains such as couscous or buckwheat as a base for vegetables or proteins, or use them in casseroles.
- Use your favourite fruit for desserts, such as chopped mangoes with a plain yoghurt or a cooked fruit with a yoghurt.
- Do not use dried fruit as it is very concentrated in sugar. Wait six weeks to include it.
- Regularly drink a glass of water plain or with lemon squeezed in it; for example, drink a glass every two hours whether you are thirsty or not.
- Use herbal tea, especially mint tea, to assist digestion.
- Include a protein twice a day such as fish, eggs, lean meat or legumes.
- Eat pasta only once or twice a week, as it will overload your pancreas (which breaks down sugar with insulin) with refined food.

- Include four to five vegetables daily – 50 per cent cooked, 50 per cent raw.

Stage three: supplementation

The following supplementation should be included in your regime when you begin the wellbeing stage (stage two).

🍀 Powdered vitamin C – one teaspoon two to three times a day for the first six weeks, then one a day for maintenance.

🍀 Vitamin B complex – this vitamin is eaten up with the overload of sugar and replacing it allows for a much more even mood and nervous system. In the first six weeks, one tablet after every meal, then one a day. Your urine may turn slightly yellow but don't worry about that.

🍀 An anti-oxidant with vitamins A, C and E to negate the free radicals in the blood from the overdose of sugar. One tablet three times a day for the first six weeks, then one or two a day. I suggest two a day if you are a sufferer of hay fever and sinus problems, as vitamin A assists and strengthens the mucous membranes in the nasal cavities.

- Herbal tea: take vervain and chamomile for the nerves, peppermint and spearmint for the digestion.

- A few cups of black or green tea are helpful as a long-term anti-oxidant.

coffee

If you are really craving coffee, have one only after food to prevent acidity build-up. Try to limit coffee to one a day. Do not have coffee if you have high blood pressure or kidney stones. Try coffee substitutes if you must: chicory or dandelion are popular.

Colourings, preservatives, additives detox

These are the really hidden pollutants that affect the wellbeing, growth and behaviour of us all, especially children.

Many people are sensitive to orange and red colourings in cordials, fizzy drinks and the lollies which we give to our children on a daily basis.

In the young, growing body, the side effects are quite visible. Within ten minutes to two hours, children can display severe mood swings, irritability, whining, temper tantrums and hitting out at the closest person possible. Sensitivity to these pollutants is often difficult to detect in the first twelve months of a child's life. I advise mothers when weaning their child to watch very carefully for abnormal behaviour when introducing a new food, especially a refined food.

When preservatives, additives, colourings and refined sugar are barred from their diets, hyperactive children improve miraculously within a week to ten days.

Read labels very carefully. For children the motto should be, 'the fresher, the better'. When they reach school years they will be exposed to swapping each others' lunches and eating miscellaneous sweets over which you have no control.

In the first four to five years, you can give them a start in refining their tastebuds to a healthy appreciation for fresh, natural foods.

This section will address two types of detox, one for children and one for adults.

Detox of children

You should not detox children under twelve. You should begin by modifying their diet – the wellbeing stage of an adult detox. It is very difficult, emotionally, for a child to change habits overnight. Slowly introducing alternative foods without colourings and preservatives is the safest, gentlest and most effective approach.

Stage one: 3 day detox

❧ Replace cordials with diluted fresh juice drinks.
  For example, use a freshly squeezed orange diluted
  with a glass of cold water.

🍀 Replace coloured (red, green, orange) lollies with slices of fresh fruit: a strawberry, an apricot or a banana. Old-fashioned honey lollies are best if the child needs to have the comfort of a sugary sweet; or fresh fruit dipped in unpasteurised honey is usually appealing.

🍀 Replace tinned food with fresh steamed vegetables (particularly for babies) and freshly stewed, home-cooked fruits.

🍀 Replace coloured fizzy drinks with peppermint- or honey-flavoured water that can be made into drinks or iceblocks. Use fresh fruit juices in a similar way.

🍀 Encourage the child to make their own sweets in the kitchen with you if they are at an appropriate age: try toffees, honey crackles and other sweets that have no additives (use honey in this case instead of refined sugar).

🍀 When at school the child will be exposed to other sweets but in my experience, a child will actually say he likes his own homemade sweets better. Encourage sharing with little friends.

🍀 Remember: always the fresher the better for the child and the adult.

Stage two: wellbeing

Follow the maintenance diet, chapter 6.

Stage three: supplementation

The following supplementation should be included in your regime when you begin the wellbeing stage (stage two).

🍀 A multivitamin once a day for children over four is advisable.

🍀 With older hyperactive children, or ADD children, a magnesium supplement has been shown to help their concentration when coming off poisons in food. Your naturopath should prescribe the dosage.

🍀 School beginners should take fish oil supplements to
assist in the development of the brain and concentration.
Give one or two capsules daily, mixed into food or honey
if they cannot swallow a capsule or dislike the taste.

🍀 A liquid vitamin B supplement for children (no added
sugars and preservatives) can be helpful to even out
children's mood swings. Check dosage with a
naturopath.

Detox of adults

It has been noticed in adult behaviour that poisons from
additives, preservatives and colourings can accumulate and
destroy many kinds of tissue including brain tissue. In short,
these toxins can disturb the chemical balance of the brain. Also,
the toxins present in these ingredients form free radicals in the
body, which can lead to forms of cancer and abnormal and
irrational behaviour. As with children, a leaky gut syndrome
often manifests.

Research carried out by Dr Alexander Schauss in the USA has
been of great interest in this area. Dr Schauss has been a pioneer in

the research of the link between hyperactivity and aggressive behaviour and diet in children since the mid-'80s. He eliminated many preservatives and food additives as well as refined sugars from the diets of schoolchildren for a period of twelve months and closely monitored the results. A large percentage of the children showed enhanced performance in school. He followed this study with another on prisoners, and similar results were found: the prisoners looked for more productive pursuits, the violence in the jail subsided and the prisoners' concentration and willingness to improve themselves increased.

We do not know yet exactly what the relationship is between preservatives, additives, colourings and sugar and depression, schizophrenia and other mental disorders. However, all the evidence so far points to a strong correlation between the presence of these toxins in a diet, and the exacerbation of symptoms of these diseases.

Stage one: 3 day detox

🍀 A three-day vegetable juice diet is ideal to remove these
   toxins and the associated free radicals from the system.

🍀 Use carrot mixed with beetroot, and a little apple if you wish to sweeten the taste. Spinach, watercress, ginger, broccoli and wheat grass juices (or combinations) are also good. All of these vegetables will concentrate on clearing toxins from the liver. Drink 300 ml of juice every two hours while you are awake. The high vitamin A and C content of this mix is critical to the internal pollutant detox. These vitamins are wonderful anti-oxidants, which are necessary to neutralise toxins in the organs, particularly the liver.

🍀 If this detox if too severe for you, then include mashed or soft vegetables, such as potato, pumpkin and broccoli, and eat a bowl full every three to four hours. Alternatively, eat two raw carrots and some raw broccoli with sticks of celery every three to four hours.

🍀 Drink water or herbal tea such as dandelion tea or chicory tea in between the juice intake.

🍀 A magnesium powder can be taken three times a day with the juice to assist in calming the nerves and helping to neutralise the effects of the toxins.

r a w   f r u i t   a n d   v e g e t a b l e s
Rich in enzymes, which are essential for the proper
functioning of our cells, raw juices of fruit and vegetables
are vital to detox and a successful maintenance program.
They should not be overlooked in your daily diet.

Stage two: wellbeing

This is quite simple.

🍀 Never use or include food colourings, preservatives or
additives, if you can help it.

🍀 Use organic produce where you can afford it.

🍀 Read all labels.

🍀 The fresher the better.

🍀 Consult the section on the liver (see pages 36–42).

Stage three: supplementation

The following supplementation should be included in your regime when you begin the wellbeing stage (stage two).

🍀 Take an anti-oxidant with vitamins A, C and E three times a day. Once you are feeling confident in your renewed vigour, usually after about six weeks, reduce intake to one a day.

🍀 Take magnesium powder or a tablet three times a day for the first six weeks, then cut back to once or twice a day.

🍀 Drink at least one to two litres of water daily.

8

Detox for environmental pollutants

CARBON MONOXIDE, pollutants from factories, unclean water from sewage wastes, poisonous sprays and chemicals from our household cleaning goods, fumes from daily inner city living, and numerous more poisons lie hidden in our environment.

We cannot control them, we can only try to combat them through fortifying our own bodies to deal with them. We can also learn what nutrients will reduce the effects of these damaging substances on our body tissues.

By acknowledging that we are existing in a polluted atmosphere, we can set about devising a daily living program that takes into account the air we breathe and the pollutants we absorb.

Blood and hair tests can give a reading on specific toxic overload in the body, especially in regard to metals such as mercury and lead. Chronic fatigue patients often find that they have been exposed to long-term toxic overload: living in an industrial area, working where street fumes are a constant hazard or even being exposed to radiation (a radiographer, for example). For these people, it is useful to know that there are clinics in Australia that specialise in chemical overload and use many methods that have worked with severe cases. This can discussed with your doctor.

Even in our home and office we are exposed to chemicals found in glues and building materials – particularly a poison called formaldehyde, which comes from particle board and causes headaches, nausea, eye irritations and respiratory problems.

Pesticides are another environmental toxin. Many pesticides promote unnaturally high oestrogen levels, which in turn have been found to promote breast and prostate cancer.

Heavy metals such as mercury, aluminium and cadmium cause a change to the DNA of the body's cells and can lead to the growth of tumours.

Lead found in gasoline and paint has been identified as a toxin in the last decade but it is still a problem in some ore smelters, lead water pipes and joints, and pottery glazes. The danger of lead exposure today lies in its combination with other toxins such as mercury. The liver finds it difficult to rid the body fast enough of this combination.

Mercury is the most toxic of all the heavy metals and the primary source of this metal is in dental amalgams. As amalgams deteriorate, mercury vapour and particles escape. Chewing can also release mercury from the amalgams. Another toxin cadmium from cigarette smoking has been found to promote the decline of lung tissue and the growth of tumours.

Anti-oxidants and vitamins

For this type of detox, we need to concentrate on the liver. We need to employ anti-oxidant foods and nutrients to clear the liver's overload. When heavy metal exposure is confirmed, a doctor can give an oral or intravenous chelating drug that binds these metals to pull them out of the blood. Read all the principles of liver and intestinal detox (see chapter 4) before you start your detox.

Vitamins C and E are the major power anti-oxidants, but there are also other anti-oxidants found in plants that can be called upon to eradicate these chemicals from environmental pollutants.

Vitamins A and C are highest in orange vegetables and fruits: carrots, oranges, mangos and pumpkin. Vitamin E is found in avocados, olive oil and oily fish. Using these foods we can develop a three-day detox to give a burst of energy and encouragement.

Green tea contains the important anti-oxidant group, polyphenols, which have been shown to be effective in preventing the growth of tumours, particularly in the lungs.

Stage one: 3 day detox

Day one

🦋 Drink one 300 ml glass of carrot juice and one glass of orange juice every alternate hour. It is best not to mix them together, as acidic fruits combined with vegetables can cause some minor digestive discomfort.

🍀 Eat raw salad made from green lettuce or rocket, with carrots and beetroot (grated if you have the time) and half an avocado. As dressing, you can use a teaspoon of olive oil and the juice of half a lemon or a dash of apple cider vinegar.

🍀 If you are hungry in the evening, make an anti-oxidant-type soup, with carrot, pumpkin, broccoli, cauliflower, onions and garlic.

Day two

🍀 Follow the same regime as day one but you may drink anti-oxidant soup as well, at two hourly intervals. Do not drink soup with the juice. Mashed vegetables (as above, with the addition of some greens such as spinach and zucchini) will be just as good as the soup if you prefer to make the preparation simpler. If you feel constipated, then include a teaspoon of vitamin C three times a day in your juice.

🍀 If you do not like pumpkin soup, then make a soup from cauliflower, broccoli, onions, turnips and garlic with just a little pumpkin. Continue with the raw vegetable salad as much as possible to spur on the liver detox and assist the gall bladder to produce bile and rid the body of toxic overload.

Day three

On day three, continue to use day two foods and begin to gently cleanse the liver by drinking dandelion tea and the herb silybum marianum (St Mary's thistle) tea.

first thing in the morning

For some people on detox, liver-clearing juices like carrot, beetroot and spinach can be just too strong first thing in the morning. If this is the case, fruit can be gentler. Soup is ideal if both of these options are disagreeable.

Stage two: wellbeing

There are no foods to eliminate in this section. However, the key is to watch what you ingest on a daily basis, to continually rid your body of the hidden and damaging effects of the daily intake of external toxins and the exposure to heavy metals and pesticides.

🍀 Eat one or two serves of orange fruits and vegetables daily; better still drink the concentrated form in juice. Have orange juice or a whole orange daily.

🍀 Drink carrot juice or eat a raw carrot daily. (You can add beetroot, a green vegetable or ginger – all have anti-oxidative value.)

🍀 Eat one avocado at least every second day.

🍀 Use cold-pressed olive oil or wheat germ oil or a mixture of both on a daily salad or vegetable serving.

🍀 Eat a variety of proteins but don't overload on meat proteins – concentrate on deep-sea fish such as salmon, cod, sardines and tuna.

🍀 Include some pulses in, for example, minestrone soup taken two or three times per week.

Stage three: supplementation

The following supplementation should be included in your regime when you begin the wellbeing stage (stage two).

- An anti-oxidant tablet one to three times a day depending on your circumstances. I recommend painters, builders, factory workers and those living in industrial areas to take higher supplements of anti-oxidants.

- Green tea: two to three cups a day, or green tea capsules: one tablet once or twice a day.

- Dandelion tea daily: it may take some time for your tastebuds to acquire the taste and it can be sweetened with honey.

- A tablet of silybum marianum once a day. This herb is also brilliant for keeping down bad cholesterol (see page 42).

- Vitamin C powder. A teaspoon once a day if you are living in an area that is high in air pollutants.

- A teaspoon of magnesium powder once or twice a day.

9

Detox for cigarettes

CIGARETTES ARE environmental pollutants we choose to inhale. This simple fact means that the habit needs special attention and understanding.

Statistics in the USA show that one-fourth of all cancer deaths are from lung cancer. (Although smoking remains the largest single known cause of cancer, the majority of cancers cannot be traced back to cigarettes. Cancer of the prostate, bone marrow and lymph nodes cannot be related to cigarette smoking, which makes us realise that there are still many tumours that can be related to many other forms of exposures to chemicals and stresses in our lives.)

If only we could see each time tobacco is inhaled what it destroys in our delicate lung tissue. The carbons build up damaging free radicals, just like those carbons we inhale unconsciously in city living.

But there are two enormous differences. We choose to smoke with a full knowledge of the side effects. We hold a cigarette to our lips and receive a concentrated burst of carbon through our airways, which destroys delicate lung tissue and cells, and breeds free radicals, which will often, in the long term, form cancers.

I don't wish to discuss the whys and wherefores of smoking, as it is a topic that could fill volumes. Let's concentrate on managing the problem: whether you continue to choose to smoke, or whether you weigh up the gains that can be achieved if you give up. If you give up, you can counteract a lot of the damage previously done.

If only one could invent a cigarette that could be very enjoyable and still beneficial to everyday living!

Many of my clients need more energy. Often they are smokers who have no intention of giving up. The interesting fact is that often I do not indicate to them that this as the main problem. Through experience, I have found that after these patients improve their energy levels through better diet and supplementation, they begin to dislike the taste and effect of cigarettes, which give their bodies a feeling of being 'unclean'.

Some clients want a full-on detox, especially if they are fed up with smoking. Others want to detox slowly, and give up over a period of time. It is different for all of us and what suits our personality is generally the right way to approach the problem.

Stage one: 3 day detox

The detox procedure here is identical to that of environmental toxins (see pages 93–95), for those who wish to give up smoking 'cold turkey'.

Stage two: wellbeing

Large amounts of vitamin C are a key factor in cutting down and finally eliminating cigarettes altogether. This vitamin is burnt out at a high rate every time a cigarette is inhaled. It is also one of the power anti-oxidants and can combat damage to the lungs. Some clients even go to their local doctor to receive injections of vitamin C, or drips in severe cases. This can be discussed with an open-minded doctor or natural practitioner.

Powdered vitamin C is far more quickly absorbed and therefore the best form to use in this case. Take at least 3 to 4 grams per day in the first six weeks. If you suffer from diarrhoea, then cut back on the dose. Always choose a vitamin C with bioflavonoids, which are substances (rutin and hesperidin) from the pith of the citrus fruits that are wonderful for treating the inflammation of the delicate tissue of the respiratory tract.

Make sure you include:

* A daily dose of a whole lemon squeezed in water with honey each morning, to help prevent the unpleasant phlegm that arises when cutting back on cigarettes.

* Anti-oxidant foods. Follow the prescriptions for the previous chapter, i.e. lots of orange juice on a daily basis for at least six weeks and then cut back to every second day.

* Fresh fish high in omega 3 and 6. It will help repair tissue. Look for salmon, cod and sardines.

* Spicy foods, horseradish and mustards, to assist in expelling mucus from the lungs and to clear the sinus passageways.

* Mint in salads: it refreshes the respiratory tract and promotes clearer thinking.

Remember also to:

- eat small snacks regularly instead of reaching for a cigarette
- clean your teeth at least every two hours, to discourage you from placing a cigarette in your mouth
- drink copious amounts of fresh, clean water to flush out toxins.

Stage three: supplementation

The following supplementation should be included in your regime when you begin the wellbeing stage (stage two).

❧ Vitamin C powder with bioflavanoids: one teaspoon in a glass of water or juice, three to four times daily.

❧ Vitamin E 500 IU once or twice a day (if you are on heart medication or blood thinners, check with your doctor regarding the dose).

❧ Salmon fish oil capsules, with omega 3 and 6, to assist in the repair of tissue. Two capsules twice daily.

❦ Vitamin B complex (make sure it includes B_1 and B_2) to prevent moodiness and assist drops in nicotine levels. One after each meal and then, when feeling better, one a day.

❦ Any organic mint tea such as peppermint, Summer Delight or ginger tea, to assist in clearing mucus from the lungs.

❦ A herbalist can provide you with a tonic made from elecampane (to assist in bringing up unwanted mucous), echinacea (to stimulate the immune system), fenugreek (to loosen phlegm on the chest), ginger (to give heat to the lungs and other areas), peppermint (to relax the lungs), avena (to blunt the cravings for nicotine), chamomile (to alleviate irritability and frayed nerves) and rosemary (to act as an anti-oxidant and a brain stimulant for memory). Combine equal parts of each herb in the tonic and take one teaspoon three times a day during this time and after for at least six to eight weeks.

This formula has worked wonders for the many clients I have helped to give up smoking.

10

Detox for alcohol

OVER THE CENTURIES, alcohol has been used for numerous reasons, not all of them detrimental to health. It has been, and still is, used as the best and finest base for carrying and preserving medicine. It was used to embalm bodies. And, of course, it has been, and still is, used for pleasure in the form of alcoholic drinks.

However, like all substances that are enjoyable, alcohol can be abused for emotional and physical reasons.

It is always best to allow a patient to write a food and beverage diary for one to two weeks, being strictly honest with what they actually eat and drink. Most people are very surprised to find they consume much more refined sugar and alcohol than they thought.

For the purpose of this chapter we will be referring only to the effects of overuse of alcoholic beverages.

In Australia, alcohol is the most abused of all the internal pollutants. It is a serious problem among young and old, male and female.

Symptoms of the overuse of alcohol are depression, moodiness, fatigue, fluctuations in weight, aggressiveness, social inconsistency, and sometimes biliousness. The feeling of being 'on the liver' may be present.

The liver is the organ most affected by overuse of alcohol. But alcohol can also have damaging effects on the joints, brain tissue, digestion and pancreas. Alcohol abuse depletes vitamin B, damages liver tissue and can cause atrophy of the brain (the wasting or degeneration of brain cells).

With the high sugar content of alcohol, the body goes into a false loss of appetite and digestive enzymes are disturbed. Many people who abuse alcohol suffer from severe nutritional deficiencies and cause damage to organs such as the pancreas, which is responsible for the assimilation of sugar. When this organ is overloaded, diabetes can occur. Joints can become wasted, meaning the integrity of the ligaments and tissue surrounding the cavities breaks down. Early-onset arthritis and other bone problems can result.

Alcohol should be drunk in moderation: I regard 'moderation' as approximately one to two glasses every second or third evening for men, and less for women (see page 113).

Red wine does contain a group of substances called flavonoids, which have been found to perform like anti-oxidants. Flavonoids are also in orange fruits. Flavonoids are known to assist the cardiovascular system and can be found in the herb hawthorn berry, which is in my Berry Tea (see page 170).

This does not mean that the more red wine you drink, the better you are, as the alcohol content still has damaging effects on the liver.

Unfortunately, wines have many additives and preservatives which, in combination with the alcohol content, can lead to toxic overload of the liver. We are all aware that alcohol damages liver tissue in large amounts, but with additives, the process can be increased rapidly (see chapter 7).

Spirits have the highest amount of alcohol and those who drink spirits on a daily basis are specifically overloading the second stage of liver detoxification. Beer and wine contain a concentrated form of sugar. The overload of refined sugar on the liver and pancreas can also cause the psychological effects prevalent in alcohol abusers.

It is interesting to note that reformed alcoholics often crave sugary sweets and chocolates when they give up alcohol, which can lead to diabetes and high triglyceride levels.

It is vital in this detox to be gentle and consistent with strict adherence to the steps. In withdrawing the body from the overload of sugar and alcohol together, we must take into account the state of the liver and the cravings for sugar. Some sugar hits can be incorporated, so as to avoid the temptation of eating total junk food, a temptation that is very common in this detox.

Stage one: 3 day detox

I recommend a semi-fast for three days on a mixture of fruit and vegetables with vitamins and herbal drinks. Fruit and vegetable juices can be used in moderation. However, it is important that we do not put any extra sugar load on the liver at this time, so it is better to concentrate on vegetables, whole fruits and quality protein.

Wholemeal rice is especially good for this detox. It is an energy-sustaining food, and takes three to four hours to break down to simple sugars. This makes it ideal for this sort of detox, when sugar 'hits' are a constant temptation.

❧ Drink one to two glasses of water with the juice of half a lemon when you rise in the morning. If craving something sweet, add a spoonful of pure honey. This assists the liver and gall bladder to get working, first thing.

❧ Make a light porridge (quite runny in consistency) for breakfast with some honey or golden syrup (no more than two teaspoons). You can use rolled oats, rice or barley porridge. This is an alkaline meal and helps to line the stomach and assists with the calming of the nervous system when withdrawing from alcohol. In fact, oats (avena sativa) are a herb, which we use as a gentle sedative and nerve rebuilder all the way through this detox stage and further into the maintenance and prevention stage.

❧ From breakfast to lunch, drink fresh orange and pineapple juice once an hour to keep the blood sugar level up.

❧ For lunch, detoxify the acid in the stomach by eating raw and steamed vegetables. The best vegetables to eat are potato, onions, turnips, and carrots, or a raw salad of greens, carrots and beetroot with avocado (no cheese). If you must attend restaurants, request these vegetables, preferably cooked in their natural state without oil or butter. Alternatively, eat raw vegetables in a mixed salad with as many different vegetables as possible: for example, lettuce, carrots, cucumber, parsley, capsicum and onions. Note: Tomatoes are too acidic in this detox.

🍀 Throughout the afternoon, drink vegetable juices. Carrot juice with added beetroot juice is best. Carrot cleanses the liver and beetroot helps to restore the pancreas and spleen. Drink a juice every hour (you may wish to add some celery, spinach and apple).

🍀 For dinner, have some soup made from root vegetables: potatoes, turnips, parsnips, onions, garlic and split peas; or, if you prefer, steamed root vegetables with the addition of broccoli and cauliflower if you like them.

🍀 Take a herbal tonic to speed up the process of detoxing liver tissue. A combination I have found good is equal parts of a fluid extract or tincture of dandelion, St Mary's thistle, artichoke, fringe tree, liquorice, chamomile and avena (oats). This can be made by a herbalist. Take a teaspoonful in a glass of water or carrot juice, four times a day for six to eight weeks.

❧ During the three-day detox and for six weeks following, some form of green chlorophyll drink (green magna or green barley) should be taken. These drinks are obtainable from health stores and help to alkalise the blood, restore the uptake of natural iron and assist in oxygen exchange in the cell tissue. Take one teaspoon, two to three times a day, added to vegetable juice or water.

Stage two: wellbeing

Continue to include in your diet all the fruits and vegetables mentioned above. It is vital to use them daily. Follow the maintenance diet, chapter 6.

It is a good idea to eat small snacks throughout the day to decrease the symptoms arising from any drop in sugar levels. You can follow the ideas for snacks in the maintenance diet.

🍀 Eat snacks of fruit between meals, and fruit and vegetable
juices with meals. If you are continually hungry, include
some protein snacks between meals such as almonds (not
peanuts as they are too much of an overload on the liver),
or tuna or salmon on bread or toast (not cheese as this is
too fatty for the liver).

Stage three: supplementation

The following supplementation should be included in your
regime when you begin the wellbeing stage (stage two).

🍀 Continue on the plant or herb tonic three to four times a
day for at least six weeks or longer if you wish. Continue
on the green magna or green barley juice two to three
times a day.

🍀 Take one vitamin B complex (B_1, B_2 and B_6) tablet after
food three times a day for six weeks and then once per day.

🍀 A mineral supplement of calcium, magnesium, zinc and
potassium will help rebalance the nervous system and

strengthen ligaments and muscle tissue. Take one tablet after each meal. If you are having sleeping problems, take two before bed, and cut out the lunchtime dose.

🍀 A fish oil capsule with salmon oil or omega 3 and 6 is ideal for the dry skin that can develop when withdrawing from alcohol. Take one capsule after each meal for six weeks and then two a day either morning or evening after food, as they tend to leave a fishy taste the mouth.

🍀 If your stomach is a little acidic, slippery elm capsules are very effective. Slippery elm lines your stomach and soaks up excess acid. Take two or three capsules before meals. If you awaken during the night with a stomach ache, take three to four capsules. Also, a calcium tablet will assist you to get back to sleep and help the acidity.

🍀 Herbal teas can be drunk to keep up fluid intake throughout the day. Peppermint, chamomile and dandelion are ideal.

🍀 Stay away from coffee and cigarettes as they stimulate the craving for alcohol.

When you are ready to return to drinking in moderation, try not to mix your drinks. I recommend for heavy drinkers that you don't consume alcohol at all for six weeks. When you resume, men should drink no more than three glasses of alcohol three times a week (nine glasses per week). Women should consume only half that. It is important to have a rest day after each day you consume alcohol. You can also take two or three slippery elm capsules before you drink to line the stomach and therefore slow down the absorption rate of the alcohol.

detox for prescription drugs and other substances

Codeine, laxatives, antibiotics and sleeping medications seem to be very common in our society and can be used to great benefit when needed. Unfortunately, in many cases, their use can be abused. Prescription and recreational drugs are abused when they are a daily habit. To detox, it is essential to substitute their use with natural herbs and preparations, or redress nutritional deficiencies with a more balanced diet.

11

Detox for your joints and muscles

PLEASE NOTE THAT this detox should not be used to treat osteo-arthritis. This disease needs to be attended to by a medical doctor, and does not respond well to a detoxification program. Hormonal and calcium supplementation can assist if monitored by your medical specialist.

Aside from the disease of osteoarthritis, many people come to me complaining of sore muscles, bad backs and aches in their joints. These discomforts are particularly prevalent in winter when the circulation is poor. A family hereditary pattern or sports injuries can also be causes.

These problems are telling us that something is not quite right in the body's system. Natural medicines can have a great positive influence, unlike the continued, long-term use of painkillers or a long course of anti-inflammatories. In some cases such as sports injuries, or the severe onset of joint or muscle pain, it is necessary to take prescription drugs. During this time you must not go on any detox regime, as you will do more damage than good. A detox should not be attempted until the severity of the attack is over and life can be resumed without drugs to help you cope. This is because the immune system in the body will already be overtaxed trying to produce white blood cells to fight inflammation, and a detox can actually weaken the body's defence systems in the short term.

Supplements can be taken alongside codeine or antibiotics to assist in withdrawal, but it is always best to check with your doctor and a naturopath. Heavier medication such as anti-inflammatories and/or painkillers such as Panadeine Forte require careful monitoring in the withdrawal phase.

The principles involved in this detox are generally quite simple. We need to begin the 'waterfall' effect. I referred to this analogy in my previous book – *The Healing Effects of Herbal Tea*. Think of your bloodstream as a river. For a river to be healthy, it needs to keep moving. It needs to have waterfalls and rapids to oxygenate the water, which in turn gives life to the flora and fauna which depend on the pure water of the river for life.

It's the same in our bodies. For good health we need to have a clean bloodstream and a moving bloodstream. This means two things:

- we need to feed our blood with healthy nutrients, and
- we need to drink enough fluids to keep the blood circulating.

In a system where the waterfall effect is working, the joints, tissues and all parts of the body are nourished and cleansed. Poisons are removed and vital nutrition is delivered to all cells to build and burn oxygen for energy and vitality.

A detox program must incorporate these principles to allow an efficient removal of the toxins that have built up over time in the cells. In removing toxins, my patients gain better mobility of joints and muscles.

These problems usually manifest in the iris. From reading the iris, I can discern an acidic constitution. This means that the individual tends to build up excess acid in their system through poor diet, a sluggish bowel or the excessive intake of refined, demineralised food. The acid often causes aches and pains in muscles and joints. (See acid and alkaline foods, pages 25–29.)

To prevent joint and muscular problems, we will look at eliminating all foods that tend to be acidic.

During the detox stage, we must neutralise the excess acid as swiftly as possible and concentrate on alkaline foods, which absorb acid and stimulate the circulation.

Stage one: 3 day detox

Day one

🍀 Drink vegetable juice all day. This can be made from carrot, celery and beetroot (40:40:20 ratio). Carrot helps the liver to detox, celery adds natural sodium, which helps water retention in the joints, and beetroot absorbs free radicals as well as stimulating the carriage of oxygen to the cells. This juice is superbly effective, so drink 300 ml every hour during the day. Drink about seven glasses of filtered water (best at room temperature for the circulation) for the day.

🍀 If you become really hungry between the juices, chew the raw version of each of these vegetables as well as rocket and watercress.

Day two

🍀 Include a broth made from celery, parsley, carrots and a few onions. Add some sweet potato if you are very hungry. You may add ginger, cayenne and garlic because they stimulate heat and circulation in the joints.

🍀 Make sure that you drink either a juice or a broth soup every hour. Water can be taken between the soup or, if you prefer, drink a herbal tea based on pure liquorice root (not liquorice lollies!). My tea, Triple E, is excellent (see page 172).

During this stage, you are continually removing acid build-up which has accumulated in the joints. You are also generally clearing away the toxic build-up which has been wearing away your healthy tissues.

Repair commences immediately, but if the detox program is followed up with the correct diet, vitamins and herbs, then tremendous relief and healing takes place.

Day three

Remain on the raw vegetable juices and broth soup but begin to introduce steamed vegetables with olive oil poured over them. The best vegetables to use are sweet potato, zucchini, cauliflower, brussel sprouts, carrots and onions. The olive oil helps to empty the bowel and lubricate the joints as well as preparing you for the adjustments in your eating habits which will maintain healthy joints.

Stage two: wellbeing

- For the next six weeks, all red meat should be taken out of the diet. The uric acid by-products from the break-down of red meat interfere with the acid/alkaline balance of the body. This acid aggravates arthritis. Red meat can be introduced back into the diet once a week once you are feeling better.

- All acidic foods should be kept to a minimum (possibly once every three days). These are: oranges, tomatoes, white sugar, refined products such as white bread and pasta, cakes and biscuits, and alcohol.

- White meats such as chicken can be eaten, but fresh fish,

especially deep-sea fish such as salmon and cod, are best because of their high levels of omega 3 and 6. These oils actually assist in lubricating the joints, just as we would oil a squeaky door!

❧ Steamed and cooked vegetables and wholemeal grains can be eaten freely. (See also acid and alkaline foods, pages 25–29.)

Stage three: supplementation

The following supplementation should be included in your regime when you begin the wellbeing stage (stage two).

❧ Salmon fish oil capsules (EPA-DHA) assist in lubricating the joints. Take one to two capsules after each meal. This dose can be doubled in winter, as cold weather can further lock up mobility.

❧ Take magnesium tablets or powder twice a day. This mineral greatly assists the alkaline balance and is essential for repair of joint and muscle tissue.

🍀 Take an anti-oxidant tablet twice a day.

🍀 A herbalist can make you up some wonderful herbal
tonics, which should be taken twice a day. Herbs to
consider are: burdock, yellow dock, guaiacum, prickly
ash, devil's claw and ginger – equal parts of each. I usually
advise that this tonic be taken three to four times daily
after soup during the detox stage (stage one).

🍀 The herb boswellia is excellent and I also recommend
an amino acid called glucosamine, which helps to
repair injured tissue and ligaments. Take one
combination tablet three times a day or one of
each twice a day after food.

🍀 A teaspoon of apple cider vinegar every morning can also
help, as it promotes the alkalinity of the blood.

🍀 Drink a carrot and celery juice daily. The juice contains
the all-important enzymes (which help the cells dispose
of free radicals), but if you can't support the taste, then
take two celery tablets daily.

12

Detox for your skin

I DON'T KNOW anybody who is not concerned about the appearance of their skin. When we are healthy, the skin has a radiant bloom that is impossible to replicate with all the make-up in the world.

Detox can improve the overall appearance of your skin, as well as treating specific skin conditions such as acne, psoriasis, dermatitis, itchiness, a sallow grey tone and fine broken capillaries that can be seen on the cheeks and nose.

Herbalists refer to toxic or poisonous blood whenever problems show externally. Where there are problems with the skin, the liver is invariably involved. This is the organ that acts as the filtering system for all the toxins that accumulate in our bodies for all sorts of reasons. Skin condition is a sure sign of the workings of our internal organs and filtering systems. If skin condition is poor, then it invariably means that the toxin filter systems in our body are sluggish. Perhaps we are not eating in a healthy way, or we are overloaded with an external pollutant; for example, pesticide sprays, air-born springtime allergies, or exposure to chemicals of some kind (see chapter 8 on external toxins). Constipation can also be a culprit, especially if it happens before menstruation, when hormones can cause an imbalance in our skin and natural detox systems.

In this chapter we will discuss the skin detox for an overload of the wrong type of food. This food does not feed the skin and cell tissue, but rather destroys it. The wrong foods can overload the immune system. This overload manifests on the skin as pustules and cysts that contain bacteria.

It is also not uncommon to see someone recently out of hospital break out in mild acne. This is usually due to an overload of prescription drugs. This is an ideal time to detoxify and it can be done safely even with the prescription drugs being taken simultaneously (see chapter 13 on hospital and surgery).

The liver is critically involved in a skin detox (see chapter 4). But repair of skin tissue is most important if you are to maintain a vibrant and healthy glow.

Stage one: 3 day detox

🍀 Drink fresh orange juice mixed with pineapple and
lemon juice hourly from breakfast to lunchtime.
These juices clear out the fatty residues in the liver
and stimulate the liver to work more efficiently in its
detoxing role. I suggest 40 per cent orange juice, 40 per
cent pineapple juice and 20 per cent lemon juice. One
tablespoon of ginger juice is also excellent to stimulate
the liver. Pineapple contains a substance called bromelian
which works as a natural anti-inflammatory, especially
for the skin and joints.

🍀 At lunchtime, prepare a large plate of raw vegetables and
drink a carrot and beetroot juice. The fibre in the raw
vegetables clears the bowel and stimulates sluggish
digestive juices. They are also filled with anti-oxidants
(these nutrients are especially high in carrots, beetroot,
onions and garlic). Other vegetables to include in this salad
are raw broccoli, radishes, lettuce and rocket. Tomatoes
should be avoided at this stage as they sometimes
aggravate skin problems due to their oxalic acid content.

❦ Water and herbal teas should be drunk frequently on this regime. The best herbal teas are: dandelion tea, red clover or Petal tea (see page 171) and Triple E tea (see page 172). Triple E contains liquorice and aniseed which work as bowel cleansers.

❦ Watermelon juice in summer is ideal, but don't mix this juice with other juices as it does not digest well with other fruits and can cause flatulence.

❦ During the afternoon, drink carrot and beetroot juice, alternating with orange juice and herbal tea. Drink one of these per hour. If you are hungry, then chew on raw food such as celery and carrot sticks with some capsicum for variety (capsicum contains high amounts of vitamin C). Note that cucumbers can cause bloating.

❦ Dinner should be a large plate of steamed vegetables, including carrots, broccoli, cauliflower, brussels sprouts, potatoes (only one or two of medium size) and spinach or peas.

🍀 Green magna juice or green barley powder are wonderful for detoxing the skin. Add a half to one teaspoon to water three times a day or mix it with your vegetable juice. Some people find the taste of the juice or powder too strong, but if you can tolerate it, it's very good for your skin. It is a great alkaliser for the blood and assists in carrying iron to the cell tissue, an essential element of skin repair.

🍀 Days two and three should be exactly the same as day one. If you are constipated at all, then include vitamin C powder: a teaspoon three times a day in a glass of water or your juice. If you feel bloated, then take a capsule of acidophilus powder before each meal and at bedtime.

🍀 The vegetables on days two and three can have a teaspoon of olive oil on them and a little vegetable salt to taste. Natural herbs from the garden such as parsley, mint, coriander and basil can be used freely.

What side effects can you expect?

Your skin may have cleared by up to 50 per cent after the three days, but you may also become worse before you improve. Often in the detox stage, the liver throws out its poisons at quite an amazing rate and the skin also throws out excess wastes initially. Do not give up. If this is the case, then I suggest taking supplements on the second and third days to speed up the detox stage. You could take the green barley powder or green magna juice, vitamin C and two anti-oxidant tablets after each meal. If you can tolerate garlic, take one to two garlic tablets after each meal, as it is a wonderful anti-bacterial herb for the skin.

Stage two: wellbeing

Follow the maintenance diet, chapter 6.

🦋 Continue to eat a raw salad each day but add protein for lunch and dinner. Try to stay away from cheese and heavy dairy products as these clog up the eliminating systems, especially the lymphatic system where white cells are made to fight infection.

Stage three: supplementation

The following supplementation should be included in
your regime when you begin the wellbeing stage (stage two).

- ❧ Include an orange and pineapple juice daily, and a carrot juice daily for at least two to three months.

- ❧ Take two anti-oxidant tablets after each meal for six weeks, and then cut back to two to four a day for the next three months. Women may need four tablets per day before a period is due.

- ❧ Drink eight to ten glasses of herbal tea or fresh filtered water daily.

- ❧ Echinacea is excellent for acne and cyst problems. I suggest two tablets per day, taken for a period of three to five months.

- ❧ One garlic tablet after each meal.

🍀 Green barley or green magna juice twice a day for
three months.

🍀 Evening primrose oil is very helpful for dry skin
conditions such as dermatitis and psoriasis. Take
one or two tablets after each meal (3000 mg per day).

13

Detox before major surgery

GENERALLY YOUR DOCTOR will give you advice on any medication you require before surgery, or any medication you need to stop. I always advise patients to stop taking vitamin E or any blood-thinning herbs a week before surgery. (Your herbalist or naturopath can advise you on details.)

A health program and minor detoxification should begin four to six weeks before a major surgical procedure (heart surgery, cosmetic surgery, knee or hip surgery or even bowel surgery).

It is important to be as fit and healthy as possible for surgery so that your body can recover as quickly as possible afterwards.

Whereas detoxing usually occurs after a certain point or event think of this detox as a cleansing of the system for four weeks prior to the event, and a building up of the immune system. Your doctor should check your iron levels (in case of anaemia) before you start.

It is also important to note here that you should not go on a strict weight-loss program beforehand, as your immune system can be detrimentally affected and the nutrients in the body, which you will need for reinforcement, can become depleted.

The following is a safe, mild detox program, which you should begin four to six weeks before surgery.

Stages one & two

Incorporate the following regime into the maintenance diet, chapter 6, so that you are in strong physical shape leading up to surgery.

- Stop alcohol four to six weeks prior to the surgery.

- Cut out all foods that contain artificial food colourings and preservatives, such as lollies, chocolates, sweet cakes, fizzy drinks.

❧ Heavy sauces, fried foods and very fatty food such as cream and cheese should also be eliminated.

❧ Keep the body well hydrated by drinking at least ten glasses of filtered water daily.

❧ Drink a freshly squeezed orange juice, and a carrot and beetroot juice daily. These assist in building healthy blood and giving you extra vitamin C boosts to keep your internal organs in optimum condition.

❧ Eat proteins such as fish, chicken, lean meat, nuts, legumes and eggs twice a day. Protein is a building block for assisting new cells and tissue regrowth.

❧ Eat as many fresh raw and cooked vegetables as possible: two to three at lunch and dinner. Vegetable and protein soups are an easy way to manage this.

❧ Include brown rice, buckwheat, couscous and other wholemeal grains to give you quality carbohydrates.

Stage three: supplementation

I suggest you discuss vitamin and herb supplements with your naturopath. It will depend on the type of surgery you require.

🐾 Make sure you are not constipated before surgery. If you are, take a natural laxative two to three days beforehand. Senna tablets or psyllium seeds husks are excellent.

14

Detox for your brain

THE BRAIN IS an organ like any other in the body. Even though it is probably the most valuable organ in our entire body, it tends to be the most neglected. We take it for granted. We tend to think that the brain feeds itself and has this magic quality enabling it to work separately from the other organs.

In many religions, fasting with or without water or food is a crucial part of a spiritual awakening. This is commendable, but in this chapter I will be referring to the principles that I believe are a safe and effective way to gain a clearer thinking brain, as well as some basic ideas to combat and counteract chemical living.

I believe that many yogis and spiritually aware people could be even more finely tuned and alert if they took more care of how they were feeding the brain physiologically. I am not underestimating here the importance of meditation, prayer and the control of our thoughts. However, I see that quality food and water are prime elements in the good functioning of the brain. Also, we do not have the privilege of living in a chemical- and stress-free world.

Detoxification is an amazing way of clearing the brain of toxins and poisons that can build up through incorrect diet and stressful living.

The feeling of toxins circulating excessively in the brain is similar to that after an alcohol overload. The brain feels foggy and heavy with, possibly, a pounding headache and sometimes blurred vision.

Just as toxins are able to pass through the wall of the intestine and bowel, so too can toxins pass through the 'brain barrier wall'. It is more difficult for toxins to do this as the mechanism of the brain is complex and has wonderful safety systems to protect the cells. It is only when there is a total overload that toxins can invade.

Chemicals that are able to do this include: ecstasy, heroin, alcohol and some pesticides. They can cause a foggy feeling in mild cases, and irreparable brain tissue damage in severe cases.

Quality fluids play a major part. Fluids are needed to bathe

the brain, help circulation and assist the removal of toxins from this organ. Water, herbal teas, raw juices and soups can be incorporated with stimulants such as ginger.

Stage one: 3 day detox

Day one

- 🍀 On awakening, drink a large glass (300 ml) of warm water mixed with the juice of half a lemon. This will help to clear the liver and stomach of poisons, which will in turn assist the detox of the brain.

- 🍀 From breakfast to lunchtime, drink a large carrot juice (300 ml) full strength. For those who find this too rich, dilute with water. Mix a teaspoon of fresh ginger either juiced or cut up finely in the carrot juice. Drink this juice every hour with a glass of water in between.

- 🍀 For those who prefer fruit, drink a large orange juice then eat one to two pieces of fruit, hourly, until lunch time.

🍀 For lunch, eat a bowl of steamed vegetables with no dressing, oil or butter. Use as many vegetables as you wish and mix the colours: orange, white and green. Do not use white or sweet potatoes.

🍀 During the afternoon, drink two to three large pots of herbal tea: Lemon Tang, Petal or Summer Delight are particularly good (see pages 171–172).

🍀 It's normal to feel a little light-headed. If it is too uncomfortable, then drink either another carrot juice or vegetable broth soup.

🍀 In the evening, drink vegetable soup with ginger or a little paprika for stimulation. Again, use a variety of vegetables as for lunch.

🍀 Continue to drink herbal tea into suppertime. If you are headachy, then go to bed on some more vegetable soup. The soup will assist in neutralising the toxins, including those in the stomach and intestine. During this time you need a lot of rest and a quiet, stress-free environment.

🍀 Repeat this first day for three to four days, varying the
vegetables to taste and using them in soup, or steamed.

Stage two: wellbeing

Follow the maintenance diet, chapter 6, highlighting the foods
above.

Stage three: supplementation

The only supplement I would advise here is acidophilus. Take two
capsules before breakfast, lunch and dinner, and before bed. This
will assist the detox of the poisons in the bowel, which in turn
help to prevent the leakage of more toxins into circulation and
into the brain.

15

Detox for nervous disorders

NERVOUS DISORDERS INCLUDE anxiety, depression, insomnia, agitation, moodiness and irritability.

Generally these are symptoms of a physical imbalance. For example, these symptoms can be associated with women with a premenstrual hormonal imbalance. These symptoms can also be associated with a drop in testosterone in middle-aged men. Also, they can be the side effects of recreational drugs or prescribed medication.

Regardless of the larger causes of nervous disorders, I have seen that a detox program and a maintenance diet can be of great assistance. In my years of clinical work, I have found that most clients suffering from these problems respond to changes in their eating habits. The symptoms appear often as a side effect of 'stressful living' and it is here that a detox can work wonders in rebuilding and repairing the intricacies of the nervous system. Those who are on the run constantly and do not take the time to eat balanced meals will often become prey to nervous disorders.

An overload of refined sugar in the diet leads to many nervous symptoms (see chapter 7). Sugar can aggravate nervous disorders, so sweet fruit and their juices should be avoided or kept to a minimum in the three-day detox program. I use soothing and nourishing vegetables and grains to 'ground' the nerves and begin to nourish the sensitive nerve fibres that have been literally 'rubbed raw'.

Stage one: 3 day detox

♣ Make a vegetable and barley soup with a few legumes and pulses. Include a wide range of root vegetables such as sweet potato and turnips. This will stabilise blood sugar levels in the body and keep the cells nourished. Drink soup at least once an hour all day. Even a small amount taken each time will continually neutralise toxins in the bloodstream that are harming the nerve cells.

Vegetables are rich in the minerals that the nerves so desperately need. They are also high in anti-oxidants, which help to clean up the poisons in the blood. Barley is classed as a mucilage grain. This means that it is soothing to the mucosal lining of internal organs including the urinary tract and the gut. This is very important for those who suffer anxiety, which is usually accompanied by a touchy, acidic stomach.

The pulses in the soup – split peas, lentils or baby kidney beans – will add protein to help regenerate nerve tissue.

🌸 Follow this regime for three days. Alternate the soup with organic chamomile, petal or lemon verbena tea.

🌸 Unlike other three-day cleansing regimes you should feel no major side effects. If you continue to feel nervous or anxious, then take more of the soup, more regularly.

🌸 If you awake in the night and feel hungry or anxious, drink a warm bowl of soup or a warm mug of milk.

Stage two: wellbeing

Follow the maintenance diet, highlighting the foods above and alkaline foods (see acid and alkaline foods, pages 25–29).

Stage three: supplementation

For those who do not include dairy products in their daily diet, it is vital to supplement your detox program with calcium and magnesium for a healthy nervous system.

16

Detox for your lungs and respiratory tract

THIS CHAPTER DEALS with problems including sinus, bronchitis, asthma, sore throats, tonsillitis, flus, colds, hay fever and conditions related to smoking (see chapter 9).

The lungs and respiratory organs are one of the most important detox organs of the body.

The stomach, liver and kidneys are major toxin eliminators; so too are the lungs. Here, oxygen is inhaled and carbon dioxide is eliminated. The quality of our sinus passageways, bronchial tubes and lungs are vital to the efficiency of this exchange. The intake of oxygen and elimination of carbon dioxide is essential to the vitality and health of every living cell in every organ in our body.

Keeping away from environmental toxins such as chemicals, carbon monoxide and, of course, smoke from cigarettes and marijuana is necessary for the health of our lungs and respiratory tracts.

Certain elements such as air pollens and pollutants from cars and factories are difficult to avoid. The maintenance diet with anti-oxidant supplements is important here, especially for those who have inherited a weakness in these major organs.

In a lung and respiratory tract detox, the aim is to cleanse the excess mucus from the airways, and to eat foods that will help protect the mucous lining of the nose, bronchioles and lungs from the aggravations of external airborne elements.

Stage one: 3 day detox

❧ Drink a glass of warm water with the juice of half a lemon and a teaspoon of raw honey first thing on awakening. The lemon helps to cut through the mucus that may have built up while lying down through the night, and the honey is a mild antiseptic and antibacterial for the lungs.

🦠 Drink a large (400 ml) freshly squeezed orange juice mixed with freshly squeezed pineapple juice (50:50) every one and a half hours. If you find this mixture too acidic, then add 30–40 per cent fresh apple juice.

🦠 In between, drink a cup of organic peppermint tea or a glass of warm water with a teaspoon of freshly chopped ginger and a teaspoon of raw honey.

You may use a pinch of cayenne powder in any of these juices. Ginger and cayenne will help carry the nourishment from the juices to these vital areas, and warm and invigorate the respiratory tract. Ginger, especially, should be placed in all the foods as much as possible.

If you prefer to eat the oranges and pineapple rather than juicing them, then do so – but make sure you eat an orange and a slice of pineapple every hour and a half.

🦠 At lunchtime, eat a raw salad filled with carrots, lettuce, cucumber, capsicum, rocket and a little tomato. Squeeze over lemon juice.

🍀 Through the afternoon drink vegetable broth (see recipe page 162) every hour and a half.

🍀 For dinner, eat a large plate of steamed vegetables. Follow with fruit after an hour and a half. Black muscatel grapes are ideal here.

🍀 Citrus juices and fruits should be used 80 per cent of the time, with black grapes and apples the rest of the time.

🍀 Hot Epsom salt baths in the evenings are excellent to speed up the elimination of toxins and excess mucus in the system. Use half a cup in the bath for adults and a dessertspoon for children from six years up. A hot water bottle on the chest for warmth and comfort in the evening is ideal too.

🍀 If you experience headaches, then eat more raw food or broth to help neutralise the toxins.

🍀 Rest is vital during this detox and it is preferable not to work.

❀ Do not stop any medication from the doctor and always take medication after food unless otherwise stated.

Stage two: wellbeing
Follow the maintenance diet, chapter 6.

Stage three: supplementation
Follow the supplementation stage for the cigarette detox, chapter 9.

17

Exercise and detox

EXERCISE IS A vital factor in keeping our bodies fit, well and free from an overload of toxins. Exercise stimulates the body in all its functions, allowing the expulsion of toxins through the skin, kidneys and bowel.

The skin is the largest organ in the elimination process as it covers our entire body and consists of minute pores that eliminate sweat and salts from our blood. Exercise stimulates elimination by increasing the heart rate and therefore blood circulation. This in turn propels both nutrients and toxins through the liver, kidneys, bowels and skin. Exercise also stimulates the endocrine system to produce the 'feel good' hormones, endorphins. It also helps in balancing our body temperature through the sweating and cooling system.

Exercise keeps our joints and muscles free and lubricated with increased blood flowing through these areas. By increasing the mobility of joints, exercise can help in the elimination of toxins from the accumulation of unwanted wastes, a problem that is evident in some forms of arthritis.

Exercise assists the laying down of calcium in our bones. This is especially important for growing children and the elderly (especially post-menopausal women) to keep bones strong.

In any form of a detox program, light exercise is advisable, such as walking daily with some stretching and meditation. This exercise is designed to put not too much stress on the body; rather, it helps in the gentle removal of toxins from the system.

When the preventive stage is reached, a heavier regime should be incorporated at least three times a week. Try your favourite sport or gym work, with yoga and stretching for the continual detoxification and toning of the body.

Saunas, steam rooms and massages

Never use a sauna or steam room during the three-day detox program. Fainting or giddiness and nausea can often result. The body does not cope well with too many extremes all at once.

Once you begin the wellbeing stage or the maintenance diet, steam rooms are a wonderful and ancient form of detoxification. Steam rooms assist in the sweating process and therefore the elimination of toxins through the pores of the skin. Plunging into a cold pool after sitting in the heat of the steam room closes the pores and assists in the circulation of the blood to the extremities such as the hands and feet.

Hot and cold variations are helpful when used after the initial detox, in the wellbeing stage. They are not to be used daily as drastic changes of temperature can weaken the body if overused. I recommend once or twice a week.

Dry saunas can be used, too, but don't become dehydrated. Water must be drunk in copious amounts before, during and after a sauna. In fact, water should be drunk frequently during all forms of exercise or detoxification.

Massage, on the other hand, is safe to use during any stage of the detox program. Massage can be extremely helpful. It assists in stimulating circulation and removing poisons from the muscle tissue that accumulate with stress and hectic living.

Epsom salt baths (using half a cup for a full-size bath) are ideal to help clean out your system on a weekly basis after completing your detox. Again, I do not recommend these baths so much during the detox program unless you are resting and not going to work. They help to pull lactic acid from the system, a toxin that accumulates in muscles during heavy exercise and alcohol drinking. Epsom salt baths are wonderful for arthritis sufferers. These baths also promote sleepiness, so always use them before going to bed, once or twice a week.

a note to sportspeople

If you are run-down with colds, flu or immune problems, it is not advisable to follow an extreme detox program of any sort, as this could further lower your immune system during this acute stage. Wait until you are out of the crisis stage of your illness and then you could follow the maintenance program for a few weeks to build you up before you do a three-day detox.

18

Minimising toxins in your environment

THE REALITY IS that we are living in a considerably toxic world. Compared with the world of our forebears, there are more people on the planet and more people crowded into our cities, and there are more toxic fumes, sprays and additives. We need to look around us and assess what we can do to minimise the environmental toxins to which we are subject every day.

We cannot set out to change everything all at once in our environment. I am also very aware that the average human being is overwhelmed by the subject: where to start, even in a simple form? My advice is to do what you can, one step at a time.

It is important to remember that our bodies are finely

designed to remove the danger of toxins, if we keep ourselves fit. We possess 'safety valves' in our eliminating organs – the liver, kidneys and digestive system – so we can tolerate a certain amount of toxic substance without any detrimental effect. The stomach and brain have inbuilt 'barriers' to prevent foreign substances passing through to our precious cells. So, for example, we experience diarrhoea after food poisoning. This inbuilt emergency system causes us some discomfort at the time, but allows us to eliminate the toxic elements very quickly.

While the body copes with toxins quite well as a physical system, it's wise to minimise the presence of toxins and chemicals around you. You will find a list following with extensive tips to help you do this. Consider this list as important, even if it takes you six months to incorporate these ideas into your everyday life with the necessities of shopping, eating and cooking.

You don't have to be extreme. You don't have to cause added stress (I have seen families blowing budgets on organic food, for example). But you certainly can, in your own way, sensibly apply some of the following:

🍀 Wash all fruit and vegetables with no skin or thin skins with an organic food wash, obtainable from good health stores. Rinse thoroughly with running water (preferably with filtered water, which can easily be attached to your tap systems).

🍀 Buy organic herbal tea, black tea and coffee whenever possible, as these products are traditionally treated with a lot of chemical sprays.

🍀 Snap-frozen vegetables such as peas and beans retain many of their essential nutrients. If you find it difficult to buy fresh vegetables daily, then this is a better option than eating worn-out old vegetables that have been refrigerated for four or five days.

🍀 Try to read labels as much as possible. Choose food with the least amount of additives; but remember that labels can be deceiving. A manufacturer can state no preservatives and additives on the label, but legally they are still able to add a certain percentage to the food. If you know you are intolerant to a particular brand, then try another that may not have the same additive that upsets you.

🍀 Certain brands of soup in tins and cartons are much better than they used to be. Many of them are free from additives and have stated use-by dates. These foodstuffs can be useful as quick snacks for yourself or your children. They are especially useful for people who do not buy food regularly and wish to keep something 80 per cent healthy in their cupboard, rather than using take-away all the time.

🍀 Tinned fish such as salmon, sardines and tuna are great items to keep in your pantry. They are excellent forms of protein, and work well when added to rice and vegetables, especially if you have had no time to shop for fresh fish. (Choose fish canned in spring water or oil).

🍀 Prepare large quantities of homemade soups (see pages 162–165) or your favourite healthy dishes to freeze in meal-sized containers. You can pull a serving from the freezer in the morning for lunch or dinner.

🍀 If you are unable, unwilling, or simply too busy to squeeze fresh juice each morning, buy commercially made freshly squeezed juices for yourself and your children. Choose juices that have very little or no preservatives. Go for colour, especially a deep rich colour similar to freshly juiced fruit. All the better if the pith part is still floating in the juice: this is high in bioflavonoids, which are essential for the prevention of influenza and alleviates bronchial conditions.

🦋 Watch your intake of alcohol. Aim for three to four alcohol-free days per week. Drink water in between alcoholic drinks, and stick to one type of spirit or wine. Mixing drinks is never a good idea.

🦋 Arrange for a water filter to be placed on your kitchen tap and use this water for cooking, tea- and coffee-making, drinking, and washing all fruit and vegetables. There are excellent water filters around. Get advice from your health food store, water shops, or even the main department stores in your area.

🦋 When buying a new home, inquire about pollution levels in the area through the local council. Look out for information about factory outlets and smog.

❀ Avoid smokers or ask them to smoke away from you.
Don't allow smoking in your house.

❀ Read information on any medication prescribed by your
doctor. Discuss the possibility of using natural methods
for the same result, or natural supplements to combat
any side effects. Your naturopath can also help with this.

❀ If you do have to take a course of antibiotics, make sure
you eat yoghurt daily, or take acidophilus powder or
tablets to replace the healthy bacteria and flora in the
bowel.

❀ Buy enviromentally friendly household detergents,
cleaning fluids and insect sprays. Some of these sprays
have caused mild to severe poisoning in pets and
children, who are at risk when playing on floors or
surfaces that have been sprayed or treated. Cockroach
traps are usually quite safe. Search for information from
government bodies or pest-control companies. Many
manufacturers are now aware of the danger of using
heavy toxins in their products. Also, research continually

proves that consumers don't like them. Look for advertising featuring the safety of products.

🍀 Floorboards in a home are always healthier than carpet, especially for those who suffer from dust mites and allergies related to the lungs or bronchial tract.

🍀 Vacuum cleaners are now available that clear dust mites from carpet.

🍀 Latex beds are excellent for back problems and are resistant to dust mites or other allergy-provoking substances.

🍀 Pillows should be changed regularly. Allergy-free pillows are worth looking into for those who suffer sinus or allergy problems.

🍀 A professional gardener can be consulted to check high-allergy plants in your garden, for those who suffer from hay fever in the spring and autumn.

🍀 Most people have changed to using unleaded petrol. If you do have an older car, trade it in for a car that can take unleaded petrol. Lead absorption is a very serious problem and, fortunately, in many countries addressed by law. Manufacturers are not allowed to put lead-based paints on the market. Cooking utensils must be lead-free. If you do have an older-style home, check your walls for remnants of lead-based paint. If your suspect this sort of paint may have been used, be extremely cautious with children and animals. They must not inhale or ingest flaking paint from the walls.

🍀 Use organic fertilisers in your garden and, where possible, make your own compost by using the remnants of fruit and vegetables. Recycling is a wonderful and worthwhile cause for yourself, your children and the planet.

🍀 Try to cut back on the use of plastics in your home. Use paper bags instead, or a string or wicker bag for shopping.

🍀 Do not go swimming at the beach after a storm. At these times, the water at suburban beaches is often flooded with effluent and run-off from sewerage and stormwater outlets. Many surfers and children acquire ear and skin infections. Wait for two to three days before swimming again.

🦋 Use cosmetics wisely and sparingly and try to find brands without too many chemicals that suit your skin. Have a few days each week without anything on your skin so it can breathe naturally. Read labels and be vigilant, especially with mascaras and deodorants that have strong chemical bases. Soaps and body lotions without alcohol and perfumes are best.

🦋 An oil burner can be used to clear the stale air in homes and offices. Eucalyptus and peppermint are especially good and other oils like lavender and clary sage assist in relaxation and stress.

🦋 Mobile phone use should be kept to a minimum until further research conclusively shows any detrimental effects.

Life after detox

REMEMBER THERE IS life after detox.

There is no quick and easy method to continued good health and those who have it are generally those who have worked hard to achieve it. It is crucial to work on factors in our everyday living to obtain the best quality of life – and the most important factors are a continued low-toxin diet and healthy environment.

I know from observing sick patients regain their health that our potential to achieve great vitality is extraordinary. I believe that a sense of vitality and wellbeing is the secret to greater happiness, more memory power, longevity, far greater energy levels, enhanced sexuality, and a sense of serenity that will allow you to open up to all levels of richness in your life.

Detox recipes

HEALTHY SOUPS AND juices are essential for a successful detox. They contain many healing properties that will help your body to regain its vitality and energy. Here are several basic recipes for soups and juices suitable for the detox and wellbeing stages. You can adjust the ingredients according to the specific detox program you are following. Warm, hearty soups are ideal in cold winter months, but in summer you may prefer to substitute fresh juices or cleansers. Or you can make a soup and enjoy it chilled. Make the most of fresh fruits and vegetables as they come into season, and choose organic products wherever possible.

Vegetable Broth

2 brown onions

3 carrots

3 sticks celery

1 small bunch of parsley

1 clove garlic (optional)

Place all the ingredients in a large saucepan and cover with 6 to 8 cups of water. Bring to the boil, then simmer for 30 minutes. Strain the liquid and drink anytime during the detox. Be sure not to consume any fresh juice one hour before or after drinking the soup, to optimise the nutrients. If you are feeling in need of extra sustenance, leave the vegetables in the broth or eat them separately.

Anti-oxidant Alkaline Soup

1 cup chopped carrot

1 cup chopped celery

½ cup chopped parsley

½ cup chopped brown onions

½ cup chopped pumpkin
  or sweet potato

½ cup chopped broccoli

½ cup chopped cauliflower

½ cup fresh or frozen peas

2 cloves garlic

Put all the ingredients in a large saucepan and cover with water. Bring to the boil, then simmer for 30–40 minutes. Add fresh herbs to taste: a bay leaf, cumin or rosemary. If you find the soup is too bland, add some chicken stock. Add extra water to make the consistency to your taste.

In winter months add turnips, zucchini, parsnip and brussels sprouts. This is excellent for anyone following the liver and bowel detox.

Cold Spinach and Leek Soup

1 bunch spinach, washed and roughly chopped

3 medium potatoes, washed and peeled (optional)

1 small bunch leeks, cut into small pieces

Place all the ingredients in a pot and cover with water. Bring to the boil, then simmer until the potato is cooked. Push the soup through a sieve. The consistency should be quite thick. This soup is excellent for digestive system.

Chickpea, Lentil and Bean Soup

1 tablespoon olive oil

2 large red onions, chopped

2 cloves garlic, crushed

1 teaspoon ground cumin

1 teaspoon ground turmeric

1 teaspoon ground sweet paprika

300 g can butter beans, rinsed and drained

300 g can chickpeas, rinsed and drained
   (or dried, if soaked overnight)
½ cup red lentils
5 cups vegetable stock
¼ cup lemon juice
1 bunch spinach, washed and roughly chopped
⅓ cup fresh mint leaves

Heat the oil in a large saucepan over a low heat, add onion, garlic and spices. Stir for a few minutes. Stir in the chickpeas, beans, lentils, stock and lemon juice. Simmer and cover for 20 minutes until lentils are soft. Add spinach for the last 5 minutes of cooking. Sprinkle with fresh mint before eating. This soup can be used for those on any detox program and during the maintenance diet.

what are pulses?

I refer to pulses as chickpeas, soya beans, lima beans, black-eyed beans, kidney beans, dried peas and lentils. Pulses are essential sources of protein and need to be included regularly in a balanced diet.

Juices

Smoothies and fresh juices make an excellent alternative to soups during the summer months. Choose one fruit or a combination, according to your tastes. For those who are not allergic to dairy products, yoghurt can be added to thicken any of the following recipes.

Fruit Smoothie

2 mangoes, peeled

1 nectarine, peeled and
stoned (optional)

1 peach, peeled

2 apricots

Place the fruit in a blender and combine. To achieve the desired consistency, use a tablespoon of yoghurt, the juice of an orange or a glass of filtered water.

Fresh Orange and Pineapple Cleanser

3 oranges, peeled

¼ whole pineapple, peeled

1 lime, peeled

1 sprig of fresh mint

Place the fruit in a blender with the mint and combine. Drink immediately.

Watermelon Cleanser

2 to 3 large pieces watermelon, chopped and seeds removed
2 sprigs of fresh mint

Combine watermelon and mint in a juicer or blender.
This juice will greatly assist the function of the kidneys
and those with poor appetite. Be sure not to consume any
other food or drink one hour before or after drinking the
watermelon cleanser, for perfect digestion. Excellent for
children or the elderly in summer.

Apple Mint Drink

2–3 apples, sliced
2 sprigs of fresh mint

Combine apples and mint in a juicer or blender.
This drink is very beneficial for a sluggish digestive system.

Apple and Pear Blend

2 apples, sliced
2 pears
1 small bunch of grapes

Combine all the ingredients in a juicer or blender. Alternate the apple and pear blend with the fresh orange and pineapple cleanser. For those on the sugar detox, this blend can be used only two to three times a day. During the sugar detox, include the vegetable broth, hot or cold, to reap the full benefits.

Banana, Papaya and Nectarine Cleanser

1 nectarine, peeled and stoned   1 banana
¼ papaya, peeled and deseeded

Blend all the ingredients in a juicer adding half a glass of orange, lime or lemon juice. Ideal for assisting bowel problems and for children as a snack

Papaya Anti-oxidant Tonic

½ papaya, peeled and deseeded   1 mango, peeled
¼ rockmelon, peeled   juice of half a lime

Blend all the ingredients in a blender and add some yoghurt if desired. Substitute any of your favourite orange fruits in this tonic, as a combination of these will give you the maximum anti-oxidant benefits.

Herbal teas

HERBAL TEAS CAN play a vital role in detoxification and preventative health. High quality fluid intake is essential as breathing pure clean air, and yet I've found that many of my clients complain of fatigue and lethargy – usually due to dehydration. During a detox program a high fluid intake is essential: and herbal teas are vital for their healing effects.

As a herbalist and naturopath, I created a range of organic loose-leaf herbal teas that would help my clients increase their daily fluid intake. I also knew that herbal teas have a marvellous influence in assisting the acid-alkaline balance of the body, which is so important in all cleansing programs particularly outlined in this detox book. These special teas assist digestion, help to soothe the nervous system, or assist in carrying nutrients around the body and excreting wastes from the blood stream.

Selecting the herb tea that is particular for your complaint is important and you may use the following guide to help you through your detox program. It is important that you continue using the herbal formulas that you like each day so that you can experience the ongoing healing effects. Herbal teas are a safe and wonderful way to maintain eight glasses of fluids daily, interspersed with raw juices and pure water.

You will often crave the herbal tea that you need for your body at different times. For example, during times of stress you may desire Petal or Apres, but when you experience acid build-up in the stomach you may crave the mint tea, Summer Delight, or a liquorice tea, Triple E. Try them as a weak tea at first and build up the taste according to your individual preferences.

🍀 **Apres** contains chamomile, fennel, aniseed and peppermint. This tea is highly suitable for those who suffer anxiety, stress, poor digestion, heartburn and mild insomnia. Chamomile has traditionally been used to soothe colic, upset stomachs in adults and frayed nerves. Fennel, aniseed and peppermint all aid poor digestion and help calm an aggravated stomach.

🍀 **Berry** contains hawthorn berries, elder berries and juniper berries. Hawthorn berry has an empirical history of assisting circulatory problems. In recent times this berry has also been found to have anti-oxidant properties. Elder and juniper berries assist the sweet taste of this natural herbal tea.

* **Lemon Tang** contains lemon grass and peppermint. This tea is ideal after fatty meals to help in the digestive process. It is cooling and soothing in hot weather and assists with kidney function.

* **Petal** contains organic red clover, lemon grass, lavender, rose petals, chamomile and buchu. This tea assists in cleansing the blood. Red clover has been used through-out history as a 'blood purifier' and now with further investigations we are seeing red clover to be a great balancer for the hormonal systems of both men and women. Lemon grass and buchu assist in stimulating the kidneys and therefore work as a mild diuretic, assisting fluid retention. Lavender, chamomile and rose petals are known to be 'calmative' plants, relaxing and healing for those who suffer stress, anxiety and general overload of twenty-first century living.

🍀 **Summer Delight** contains organic spearmint, peppermint, lemon grass and aniseed. This minty tea is ideal for
assisting the detox process of the digestion by stimulating
digestive enzymes and relaxing and calming the body.
Peppermint has a long history of aiding fish and meat
dishes in the digestion process and this tea is ideal after
any meal.

🍀 **Triple E** contains liquorice root, aniseed, fennel and
peppermint. This tea has a profound healing effect on
the bowel and stomach, helping with sluggishness and
heartburn. Through history the healing effects of the
pure liquorice root as a mild anti-inflammatory are well
know. Hence liquorice is used in most cough medicines
and laxative type medication.

For optimum detoxifying results from these herbal teas, wait
until the tea has cooled to room temperature before drinking.

Acknowledgements

I would like to thank Executive Publisher Julie Gibbs, who made this book possible by inspiring me to write on this vital subject. Secondly, my writing assistant Catherine Hanger, who helped me untiringly to give shape to my ideas. And my editor Kirsten Abbott, who has the sweetest and kindest way of understanding my writing and shaping the contents to make this book so readable and practical.

I would also like to thank the Mediherb and Health World for their invaluable assistance in providing essential information.

But most of all I would like to thank my late parents for encouraging me to write on the subject I love and for always being my greatest fans.

Bibliography

Baker, Sidney MacDonald, M.D., *Detoxification and Healing*, with a foreword by Jeffrey S. Bland, Ph.D., Keats Publishing Inc., New Canaan, Connecticut, 1997.

Bennett, Peter, N.D. & Barrie, Stephen, N.D., *7-Day Detox Miracle*, with a foreword by Jeffrey S. Bland, Ph.D, Prima Health, Rocklin, California, 1999.

Bland, Jeffrey S., Ph.D., *The 20-Day Rejuvenation Diet Program*, with Sara H. Benum, M.A., Keats Publishing, Los Angeles, California, 1997.

Bone, Kerry, *Liver Detoxification and Plants*, Mediherb Pty Ltd, from a lecture given 15 March 1997 in Australia.

Bragg, Patricia, Ph.D. & Bragg, Paul, N.D, Ph.D., *The Shocking Truth About Water*, Health Science, California, USA, 1990.

Calbom, Cherie & Keane, Maureen, *Juicing For Life*, Avery Publishing Group Inc., Garden City Park, New York, 1992.

Dengate, Sue, *Fed Up*, Random House Australia Pty Ltd, Sydney, 1998.

Lyon, Michael R., M.D., *Healing the Hyper Active Brain: Through the New Science of Functional Medicine*, Focused Publishing, Calgary, Canada, 2000.

Osiecki, Henry, B.Sc. (Hons), *The Physicians Handbook of Clinical Nutrition*, Biocepts Publishing, Queensland, 1994.

Perlmutter, David, M.D., *Brainrecovery.com: Powerful Therapy for Challenging Brain Disorders*, with a foreword by Bernie Siegel, M.D. and Jeffrey S. Bland, Ph.D., The Perlmutter Health Center, Naples, Florida, 2000.

Sapolsky, Robert M., *Why Zebras Don't Get Ulcers. A Guide to Stress, Stress Related Diseases, and Coping*, W.H. Freeman and Company, New York, 1997.

Steingraber, Sandra, *Living Down Stream*, Addison-Wesley, Massachusetts, 1997.

Index